LONG-TERM AMBULATORY ELECTROCARDIOGRAPHY

DEVELOPMENTS IN CARDIOVASCULAR MEDICINE

VOLUME 20

Series ISBN 90-247-2336-1

LONG-TERM AMBULATORY ELECTRO- CARDIOGRAPHY

edited by

J. ROELANDT, M.D. and P.G. HUGENHOLTZ, M.D.

Thoraxcentre, Erasmus University,
Academic Hospital Dijkzicht,
Rotterdam, The Netherlands.

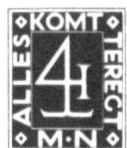

1982

MARTINUS NIJHOFF PUBLISHERS
THE HAGUE/BOSTON/LONDON

Distributors:

for the United States and Canada

Kluwer Boston, Inc.
190 Old Derby Street
Hingham, MA 02043
USA

for all other countries

Kluwer Academic Publishers Group
Distribution Center
P.O. Box 322
3300 AH Dordrecht
The Netherlands

Library of Congress Cataloging in Publication Data ⏾
Main entry under title:

Long-term ambulatory electrocardiography.

(Developments in cardiovascular medicine ;
v. 20)
Proceedings of a symposium held Oct. 1981
at the Thorax centre of the Academic Hospital
Dijkzigt and the Erasmus University, Rotterdam
sponsored by the European Society of Cardiology.
Includes index.
1. Electrocardiography, Ambulatory--Con-
gresses. 2. Heart--Diseases--Diagnosis--Con-
gresses. I. Roelandt, Jos. II. Hugenholtz,
P. G. III. European Society of Cardiology.
IV. Series. [DNLM: 1. Electrocardiography--
Methods. 2. Arrhythmia--Diagnosis.
3. Monitoring, Physiologic. W1 DE997VME v. 20 /
WG 140 L849]
RC683.5.A45L66 1982 616.1'207547 82-8042
ISBN 13:978-94-009-7572-9

ISBN-13:978-94-009-7572-9   e-ISBN-13:978-94-009-7570-5
DOI: 10.1007/978-94-009-7570-5

PREFACE

Recent technological developments have brought long-term ambulatory electro-cardiography to the front of clinical cardiology. Its application for solving clinical problems potentially related to cardiac arrhythmias is rapidly increasing.

In the meantime, the method has found widespread use in the identification of patients at risk for cardiac death as well as in the assessment of therapeutic interventions.

It was the purpose of this symposium to bring together an international group of authorities in order both to provide an overall view of the field and to discuss critically the value of clinical, epidemiological and research applications of long-term ambulatory electrocardiography in the light of new concepts and recent advances.

The first section of this volume discusses the methodology and the performance criteria of the equipment and analysis systems.

In the second section, the potentials and problems encountered in the use of long-term ambulatory electrocardiography for solving clinical questions and for predicting the occurrence of clinically important arrhythmias are extensively dealt with. New applications such as continuous ST segment monitoring, blood pressure measurement and other physiologic parameters are also included.

Prevalence variability and prognostic aspects of ventricular arrhythmias, both in normals and in patients with cardiac disease, are the subject of section 3. The last section provides a critical review of the use of the method for the evaluation of therapeutic interventions with drugs. The editors feel that this volume represents the 'state of the art' in this newly important area of clinical cardiology.

J. Roelandt
P.G. Hugenholtz

ACKNOWLEDGEMENTS

The contents of this volume represent the accumulated scientific information that emerged from the symposium on Holter Electrocardiography held in October 1981 at the Thoraxcentre of the Academic Hospital Dijkzigt and the Erasmus University in Rotterdam.

Each of the speakers kindly consented to supply a manuscript of their presentation and we would like to express our gratitude to them.

The symposium was sponsored by the European Society of Cardiology and financial support was provided by the Cardiolab Foundation.

The organization required a great deal of work and of secretarial assistance. Mrs Marjolijn Sneep-de Korver handled this with great dedication and efficiency, for which we are most grateful. We also much appreciate Mr B.F. Commandeur's professional help with the production of this volume.

J. Roelandt

January 1982   P.G. Hugenholtz

CONTENTS

SECTION 3. EPIDEMIOLOGIC AND PROGNOSTIC ASPECTS OF VENTRICULAR ARRHYTHMIAS

SECTION 4. VALUE OF LONG-TERM AMBULATORY ELECTROCARDIOGRAPHY IN THE EVALUATION OF THERAPEUTIC INTERVENTIONS FOR THE PREVENTION OF PREMATURE CARDIAC DEATH

CONTRIBUTORS

Bachman, K., Herzzentrum der Universität, Ostl. Stadtmanerstrasse 29, 8520 Erlangen, BRD.

Bethge, K.P., Medizinische Hochschule Hannover, Abteilung für Innere Medizin, 3 Hannover-Kleeveld, BRD.

Burckhardt, D., Division of Cardiology, University Hospital, CH-4031, Basel, Switzerland.

Connolly, S.J., Cardiological Division, Stanford University, Stanford, CA 94305, USA.

Coumel, P., Department de Cardiologie, Hôpital Lariboisière, 2, Rue Ambroise Paré, 75010 Paris, France.

Curry, A., Guy's Hospital, Department of Cardiology, St. Thomas Street, London SE1 9RT, United Kingdom.

Durrer, D., Department of Cardiology, Wilhelmina Gasthuis, 1e Helmerstraat 104, 1054 EG Amsterdam, The Netherlands.

Glogar, D., Kardiologische Universitätsklinik, Garnisongasse 13, A-1097 Wien, Austria.

Graboys, T B. Harvard University, School of Public Health, 665 Huntington Avenue, Boston MA 02115, USA.

Hoffman, A., Division of Cardiology, University Hospital, CH-4031 Basel, Switzerland.

Joskowicz, G., Kardiologische Universitätsklinik, Garnisongasse 13, A-1097, Wien, Austria.

Jost, M.V., Division of Cardiology, University Hospital, CH-4031, Basel, Switzerland.

Julian, D.C., University of New Castle, Freeman Hospital, New Castle-Upon-Tyne, NE7 7DN, United Kingdom.

Kaindl, F., Kardiologische Universitätsklinik, Garnisongasse 13, A-1097, Wien, Austria.

Klein, H., Medizinische Hochschule Hannover, Abteilung für Innere Medizin, 3 Hannover, 3 Hannover-Kleeveld, BRD.

Kulbertus, H., Université de Liège, Hôpital de Bavière, 66, Boulevard de la Constitution, 4000 Liège, Belgium.

Leclercq, J.F., Hôpital Lariboisière, 2 Rue Ambroise Paré, 75475 Paris, France.

Lubsen, J., Thoraxcenter, Erasmus University, P.O. Box 1738, 3000 DR Rotterdam. The Netherlands.

Luetold, B.E., Division of Cardiology, University Hospital, CH-4031, Basel, Switzerland.

Manger Cats, V., Department of Cardiology, Wilhelmina Gasthuis, 1e Helmerstraat 104, 1054 EG Amsterdam, The Netherlands.

Moss, A., 873 Elmwood Avenue, Rochester, NY 14620 USA.

Okkerse, R., Thoraxcenter, Erasmus University, P.O.Box 1738, 3000 DR Rotterdam. The Netherlands.

Prineas, R., University of Minnesota, Laboratory of Physiological Hygiene, School of Public Health, Stadium Gate 27, Minneapolis MI 55455, USA.

Ripley, K.L., Thoraxcenter, Erasmus University, P.O.Box 1738, 3000 DR Rotterdam, The Netherlands.

Rodriquez, I., Cardiological Division, Stanford University, Stanford CA 94305, USA.

Simoons, M.L., Thoraxcenter, Erasmus University, P.O. Box 1738, 3000 DR Rotterdam, The Netherlands.

Slama, R., Hôpital Lariboisière, 2 Rue Ambroise Paré, 75475 Paris, France.

Sleight, P., Oxford University, 32 Crown Road, Wheatley, Oxford, United Kingdom.

Steinbach, K.K., Kardiologische Universitätsklinik, Garnisongasse 13, A-1097 Wien, Austria.

Weber, H., Kardiologische Universitätsklinik, Garnisongasse 13, A-1097 Wien, Austria.

Winkle, R.A., Cardiological Division, Stanford University, Stanford CA 94305, USA.

Zeelenberg, C., Thoraxcenter, Erasmus University, P.O. Box 1738, 3000 DR Rotterdam, The Netherlands.

HOLTER MONITORING – HOW SHOULD IT BE PERFORMED?

P.V.L. CURRY, MD, MRCP.

Essential to the diagnosis and management of paroxysmal episodes of cardiac arrhythmia and ischaemia is electrocardiographic documentation. Continuous 24 hour ECG recording or a similar continuously available telemetric or transtelephonic ECG recording satisfies this need.

A vital requirement is that such systems faithfully capture, recognise, process and reproduce those abnormalities that threaten life or cause important haemodynamic disturbances. Such systems must record specifically profound bradycardias, tachycardias and ischaemia. In the future, they will be required to reproduce less severe abnormalities of cardiac electrophysiology including minor atrial arrhythmias and minor stigmata or localised partial thickness ischaemia.

One might conclude, in general terms, that continuous electrocardiographic monitoring systems must provide perfectly recorded, continuous, simultaneous 12 lead ECG's of unlimited duration for export analysis, (assisted only where completely reliable by automation), and should include an input from the patient in terms of symptoms and activity by careful instruction and rehearsed co-operation if the final amalgam of data is to be of maximum clinical value. Let's examine this preliminary conclusion in more detail.

In preparing perfect recordings, collection of the biological signal must be optimum. Artifacts must be minimised at source and throughout processing. Undoubtedly the patient-lead-interface is critical and requires no further emphasis. Each department develops its own method of lowering the impedance at this interface and some have tried sub-dermal electrodes although pain at the site of implantation often becomes significant after 12 hours with this technique that otherwise provides the best signals. Further work is required in this field. Operators are aware of artifacts produced by the recording leads and their interface with the recorder, monitor artifacts, artifacts in the replay unit and throughout the system to the final ECG printout. The entire 24-hour ECG should meet AHA requirements in its final printout format. Calibration at the onset of recording is essential and the effect of specific physical manoeuvres on ECG appearances is also best indicated at this stage, (lying, deep breathing, bending etc. can be indicated by appropriate use of the event-marker and an event-marker code).

More time should be spent in instructing the patient specifically in awareness of symptoms of interest, use of the event-marker and completion of the diary. Many clinical studies have demonstrated the poor relationship between patients' symptoms on the one hand and recorded ECG abnormalities on the other. How much of this discrepancy is due to our own failure to adequately prepare our patients' participation?

Recorders must be light and in every other respect acceptable to the patient, (appearance, low noise production etc.). Recorders should impart an independent unique time code to the tape for subsequent accurate event localisation as is now available, e.g. in the new Tracker recorder, (Reynolds Medical). The recorders should accept multiple ECG channels since all electrocardiographic abnormalities have a vector and arise from various sites on different occasions. This applies both to ECG manifestations of ischaemia as well as cardiac arrhythmias and the ideal would be the provision of a continuous 12 lead ECG. Physicians accepting one, two or four channels must ask themselves why they ask for a full 12 lead ECG in their routine cardiac clinics?

A debate persists regarding optimum requirements for recorders applied to the detection of cardiac ischaemia. Recently FM recorders have been considered to be more accurate for such ECG manifestations that predominantly affect the low frequency range of the spectrum, (usually DC to 30Hz). Ischaemia can be reliably detected by such recorders as represented by 1 mm. depression of the ST segment, (Medilog 2 recorders. Oxford Medical Systems Ltd.). Some of the newer AM recorders are now also promoted as providing this facility but older models are less reliable and can both fail to detect and even worse, exaggerate cardiac ischaemia. Indeed, they may even artificially create appearances suggestive of cardiac ischaemia. Once again, multiple ECG channels are essential during such recordings and in our experience, the positions shown in figure 1 relate to important regions of the 12 lead ECG, (figure 2).

How reliable is automatic processing of the 24 hour recording? Can we trust the diagnostic accuracy of available systems? If they fail to detect life threatening cardiac arrhythmias or profound episodes of ischaemia when entrusted with the task, they are not only worthless but dangerous. Yet, in fairness, certain arrhythmias defy accurate classification by the most expert cardiologist and we must not expect systems to achieve more than our own limited capacity for electrocardiographic deductive interpretation. A wide QRS complex tachycardia is a classical example of such limitation although we might expect a system in the future to scan for fusion beats and independent P wave activity to assist likely diagnosis. The detection between sinus bradycardia on the one hand and complete heart block on the other producing a ventricular rate of 35 bpm is made by analysis of P wave activity, so surely we can expect automation to encompass this facility in the future. Probably it will mean teaching an analogue pattern at the onset of analysis based on P wave appearances in perhaps four channels simultaneously. It is remarkable in this context to note the development of a permanently implantable pacemaker, (Mirowski et al. 1981), that reliably detects not only

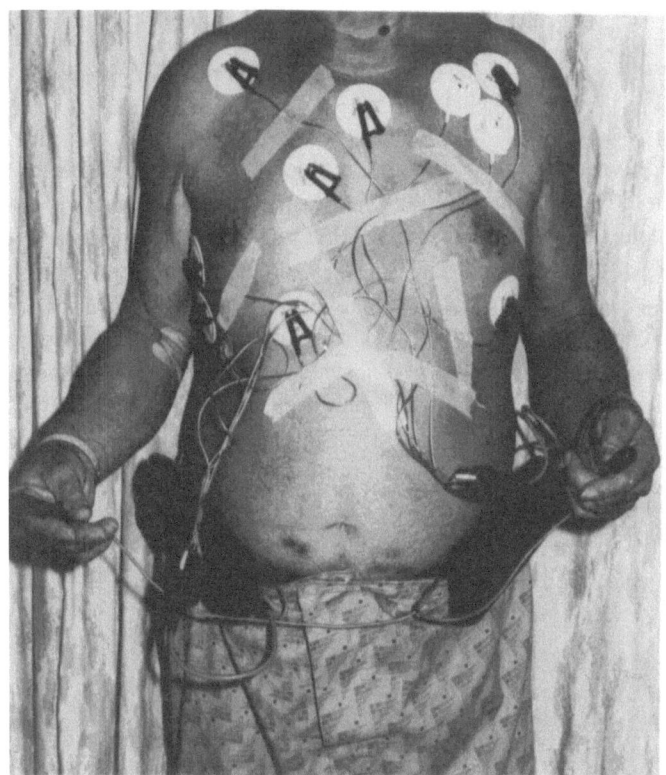

Figure 1. Multi-channel lead positions for FM recordings.

RESTING 12 LEAD ECG WITH AMBULATORY TRACINGS INTERPOSED.

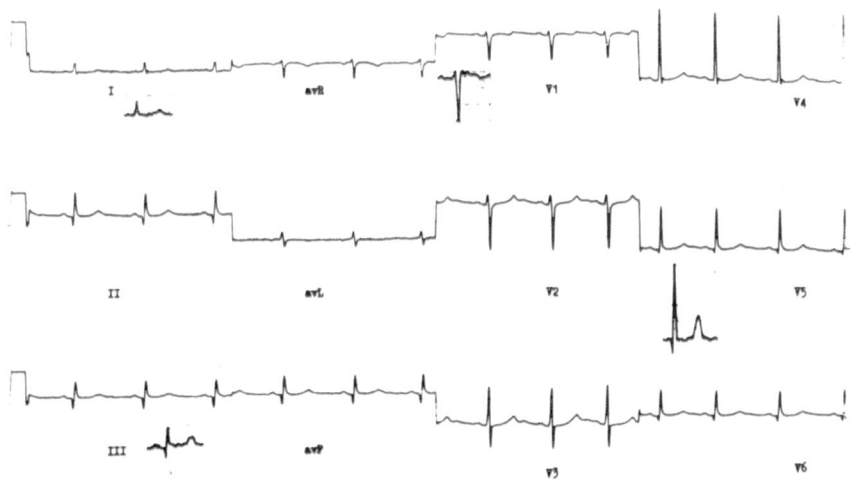

Figure 2. Four bipolar ECG's (inset) equivalent to standard Leads 1, 3 and to Leads V1 and V5.

4

bradycardia for demand ventricular pacing, but also ventricular fibrillation for internal defibrillation. Surely the latter principle can be applied to detection of atrial fibrillation with appropriate analogue teaching of atrial normality, combined with ventricular blanking and separate analysis.

There is a growing use of special pacemakers both for physiological and anti-tachycardia pacing. Often an assessment of efficacy or documentation of suspected faults requires 24-hour ECG recording. Our automatic analysis systems must keep pace with these complex ECG patterns created by such new pacing systems. Analysis of the pacing artifact is an addition to the requirements already outlined above for the analysis of tachycardias and bradycardias, and logic algorithms must be developed to examine the relationship between such artifacts and natural events to assess the function of the pacing system as a whole. At all times the expert must apply his experience to the sophisticated analysis and I doubt we shall ever be able to dispense with operator over-view for most accurate analysis. We may be able to assist ourselves in this task by more comprehensive use of the teaching phase at the onset of an ECG analysis.

A display of the analysis has to be meaningful. Seeing is believing. There are immediate advantages in condensed display of the entire ECG, (figures 3A and 3B), but at the moment, this facility is expensive – almost prohibitively so.

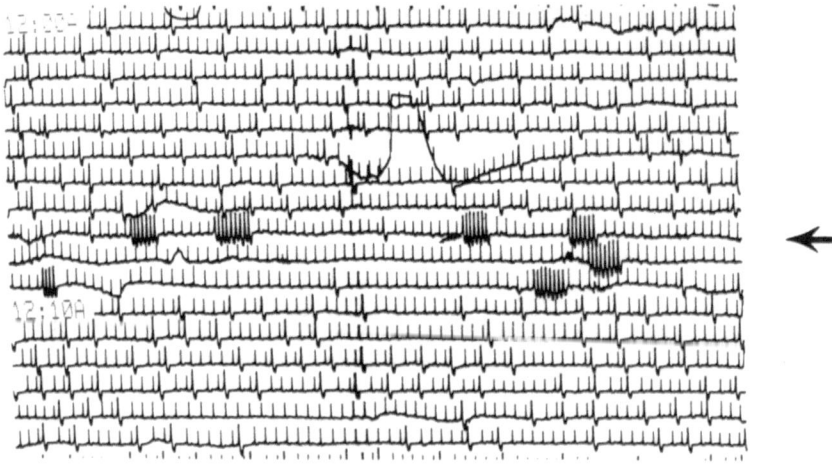

Figure 3A. Obvious salvos of wide complex tachycardia.

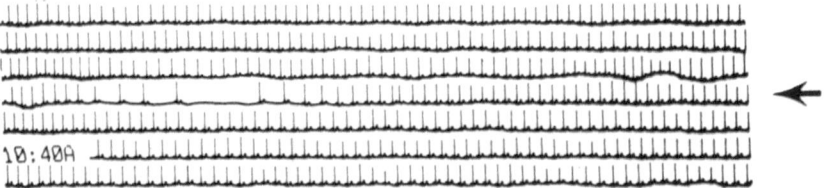

Figure 3B. An evident episode of bradycardia.

Alternative techniques of display make use of histograms but these may fail to create the same clinical impression as does the real signal. Their use in research comparisons and quantification however is irreplaceable and as always, both display facilities have a part to play depending on requirements. Episodes of ST segment depression or elevation can be well represented on trend recordings and displayed against simultaneous changes in heart rate with implications for mechanism of ischaemia and treatment of such mechanisms. Simultaneous availability of the real time ECG however emphasises the abnormality and assists interpretation of the trend.

Our second conclusion may therefore be that the level to which automation is used in the analysis and display of the recorded data is determined by clinical or research needs.

New Developments

Multi-channel long distance telementry is now available. Transtelephonic monitoring is also being developed. Furthermore, since there is a need for a prolonged period of recording to capture an infrequently occurring paroxysmal disorder of either cardiac arrhythmia on the one hand or ischaemia on the other, long play cassette recorders are being developed, (e.g. the Cardiocassette 10 Day Recorder. Reynolds Medical). Doubtless, we shall see new electronic technology applied to permit prolonged ECG recording, perhaps even to the extent of incorporating "bubble memories".

Reference

1. Mirowski M, et al. Am.H.J. 102, no. 2, pp. 265 to 270, 1981.

EQUIPMENT SPECIFICATIONS AND PERFORMANCE CRITERIA: CLINICAL EVALUATION

CEES ZEELENBERG, KENNETH L. RIPLEY, RUURD OKKERSE

The range of Holter analysis equipment on the market extends from the simple hardware scanner, which basically counts the beats on a tape and reports incidence of simple arrhythmias (premature beats, sinus arrest) to the complex (and expensive) computer systems with multiple users, sophisticated arrhythmia detection and elaborate editing facilities. Selection of the most suitable equipment for a given installation will depend on a number of factors, of which price, personnel requirements and workload are likely to be the most critical today. Whatever the constraints these basic factors may place on the initial requirements, it is essential to initiate the selection process by defining clearly the functions required of the system. One of the most basic questions that must be asked is 'what percentage of the work is clinical and what percentage research (if any)', in order to be able to give a proper weighting to requirements for facilities not usually needed in straightforward clinical work, such as accurate PVC counts or an extensive database. It is also essential to determine whether or not there will be any administrative work to be automated at the same time. Once these factors have been laid down, the clinical requirements of the system can be specified in terms of reporting facilities and type of analysis (e.g. 'ST-T segment analysis needed', 'PVC counts required'). Finally, there will often be technical or clinical-technical constraints (e.g. 'frequency response desired', 'accuracy of PVC detection). Once all these factors have been identified and suitably weighted, it is possible to select a shortlist of candidate systems for further review.

At this stage the following points should also be considered. Firstly, some quantitative measure of system performance in clinical terms with respect to the required clinical functions is important. Secondly, and perhaps the most essential of all, the user friendliness and ergonomic aspects of the system should be evaluated, with due attention being paid to the views of the staff who will operate it. Thirdly, such technical aspects as system response, capacity and extensibility should be considered. In many institutions it will also be necessary to look at compatibility with existing systems and, possibly, at communications facilities. Last, but not least, system reliability and manufacturer support, documentation and maintenance should play a considerable role in the selection process.

Naturally, it is quite possible that no system will fulfil the requirements since, in practice, every system, regardless of price, is a compromise. There are really only three options open if this happens: to relax the requirements (read price/performance), to modify available equipment (inhouse, through the supplier or through a third party) or just wait in the hope that next year's model will be better.

As mentioned earlier, performance measures are an important part of equipment selection. They can be broadly divided into two categories: a static performance measure or system evaluation, which is typically carried out in order to compare different systems and to quantitate the performance of a particular system; and a dynamic measure or quality control which should be performed regularly for each production system to monitor its performance for individual tapes.

The most extensive work in the area of system evaluation has been carried out for ventricular arrhythmia detectors, probably due to common interest here between coronary care monitoring and ambulatory monitoring. Evaluation is especially relevant in this area because the scanning equipment usually includes a relatively expensive computer system as an important component. Prices of this type of equipment vary widely, and are not necessarily linked to the detector performance. Ideally, an evaluation should use all possible ECG data in order to expose every problem in a detector. Since such a test is impossible, a subset must be selected in the hope that the results will be representative. The most appropriate method of formally testing and comparing arrhythmia detectors is to select some large but manageable set of data which contains sufficient variety to expose most weaknesses and then to test each detector on the same data. Two groups, in particular, have contributed heavily towards solving this problem. In September 1972, the Evaluation Group for Arrhythmia Detectors (EGAD) (1) was formed with the goal of creating a database with beat by beat annotations to be used as a "Gold Standard" for system development and evaluation purposes. The AHA was asked to sponsor this effort. In 1977 a full contract proposal was subsequently submitted by the AHA to the National Heart, Lung and Blood Institution, which was approved and funded. The database has since been implemented at Washington University in St. Louis, in conjunction with many institutions all over the world, and will soon be available for distribution (2). Meanwhile, Massachusetts Institute of Technology (MIT) in conjunction with Beth Israel hospital in Boston, has built a similar database (3), compatible in design with the AHA, which has been available since 1980. Although broadly compatible, these two databases differ in size, provenance of data, sampling frequency, length and degree of annotation. Both databases are intended for testing ventricular arrhythmia detection rather than general arrhythmia analysis. Each type used (MIT 48, AHA 160) has two channels of sampled data with 12 bit accuracy, the MIT tapes are sampled at 360 samples/sec and the AHA ones at 250. The MIT tapes are half an hour long, the AHA ones are three hours. Beat by beat annotations are provided for the whole of each MIT tape and for the last half hour of each AHA one,

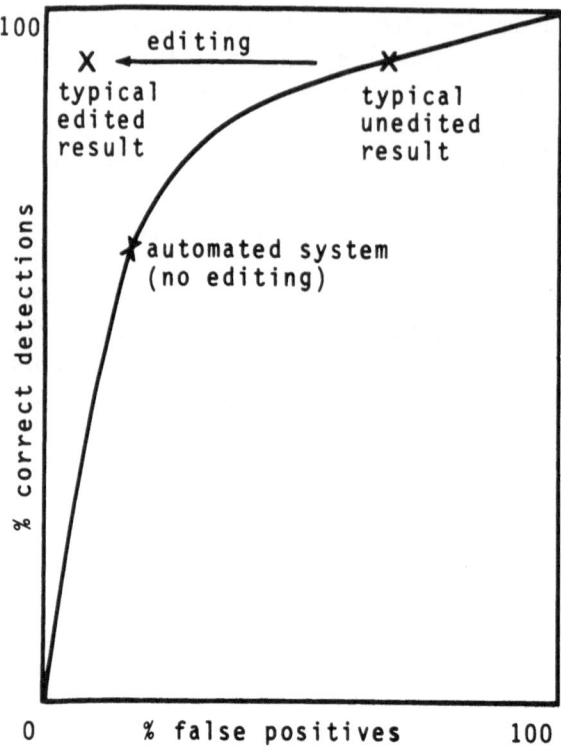

Figure 1. Receiver Operating Characteristics (ROC) illustrating detector performance.

showing time of occurrence of each beat together with a label indicating beat type (beat of non-ventricular origin; premature ventricular contraction – PVC; ventricular escape beat; fusion beat; R-on-T; paced beat; indeterminate origin; unreadable; onset and offset of ventricular fibrillation or flutter; for MIT only, supraventricular premature contraction – SVC). The underlying rhythm is also documented. The MIT set of 48 tapes comprises local data only, half being selected randomly from the routine clinical population and half being specially chosen for the problems they display. The AHA database, on the other hand, comprises 160 tapes obtained from a range of institutions and divided into eight arrhythmia classes (no PVCs; isolated uniform PVCs; isolated multiform PVCs; bigeminy; R-on-T; couplets; ventricular tachycardia; ventricular fibrillation), making it possible to test or optimise a detector for one specific arrhythmia. The whole database has been partitioned into a test set and a development set. The latter will be available to system developers and users but exact rulers for the distribution of the test set have not yet been formulated.

In practice, the availability of such a database only partially solves the problem of measuring and comparing the performance of different arrhythmia detectors. Further problems arise in the different system approaches used in these detectors. Some work fully automatically, i.e. without human intervention, while others

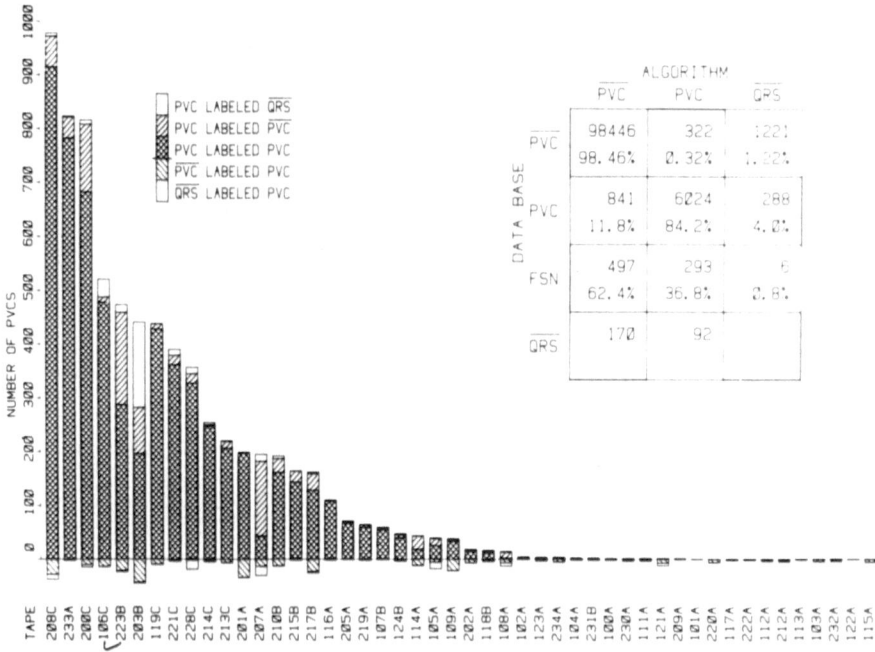

Figure 2. Evaluation Results Arrhythmia Detector using MIT/BIH Database.

depend on the skills of a human operator and a third category has a fully automatic pass followed by selective overreading by an analist. It is obvious that in the last two cases the overall performance does not only depend on that of the computer system, but also on the skills of the operator.

The effect of human interaction on system performance may be illustrated by means of the Receiver Operating Characteristic (ROC). Figure 1 shows an example of this. The ROC curve shows the basic trade-off that always has to be made between false-positive and false-negative detection: here a high detection rate results in many false positive PVCs, while a low false positive rate is at the cost of a low detection rate. The optimum working points are usually found just under the 'elbow' of the curve. A fully automatic detector with fixed criteria may be set to yield the operating point shown. Adding operator intervention during the classification process allows the detector to achieve a better working result. When, for instance, an operator checks all beats labeled PVC, virtually all false positive PVCs may be eliminated. This approach is usually combined with an initial setting for a high detection rate (and high false positive rate), so that the combined result yields both a high detection rate and a low false positive rate, although this may be at the cost of a lot of operator time.

Another pitfall in the evaluation process is caused by the wide variation in results found with any given detector over a range of tapes. Figure 2 shows the evaluation results of a particular algorithm tested using the MIT database. Tapes

N_A = total number of PVC's in testtape

N_C = total number of correct PVC detections in testtape

average detection ratio $A_{mean} = \overline{N_C/N_A}$

gross detection ratio $A_{gross} = \Sigma N_C / \Sigma N_A$

estimate detection ratio A_{est}

Median detection ratio A_{median}

Same database and detector:

A_{median} = .92

A_{gross} = .87

A_{mean} = .76

A_{est} = .72

Figure 3. Performance Measures Arrhythmia Detector.

have been ranked in order of decreasing PVC activity. It can be seen that any attempt to summarise such a result in one, or two, numbers (e.g. sensitivity and specificity) may not give a very useful measure of the overall performance of a detector when used for comparison purposes. Figure 3 further illustrates this problem by showing various ways in which a single parameter, the PVC detection ratio, may be calculated and the very differing numbers obtained for the same set of results using the various methods. The values obtained for the tapes and algorithm used in the previous example range from the 'median detection ratio' of 92% to the 'estimate detection ratio' (based on a mathematical model of this type of system) (4) of 72%.

The second main theme of this paper, quality control, will be discussed in the specific context of the routine use of a complex, computer-based Holter analysis system, although the techniques used are applicable (with some modifications perhaps) to the whole range of system types from simple scanner up. However, the poorer the facilities of the system, the more operator time will be required to perform quality control testing. Quality control is here considered as the regular sampling of the input and output streams in order to determine the accuracy of the system as a whole (equipment plus operator). A major byproduct of quality control methods tends to be the provision of management statistics to be used in optimising system performance and planning resource allocation. The discussion will be illustrated with some practical results obtained from the system at the Thoraxcentre in Rotterdam. Before describing either techniques or results it is perhaps useful to describe the system layout briefly. The Thoraxcentre in fact

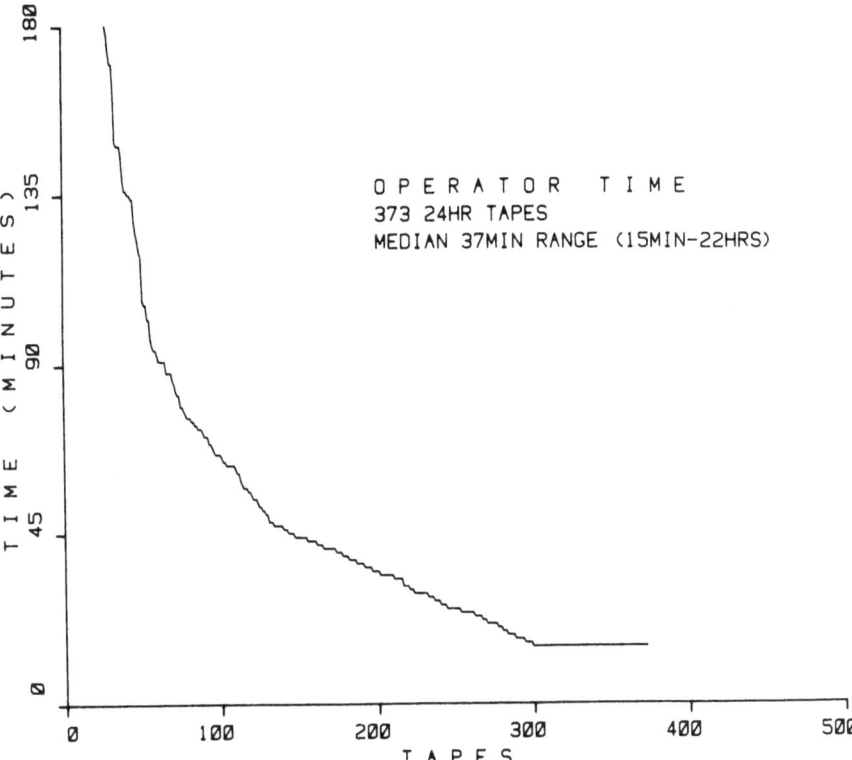

Figure 4. Editing Time.

uses two processing facilities: commercial scanning equipment used for some research and for all routine clinical work (90%) of total load and an ARGUS high-speed tape scanning system (centred on a fair-sized minicomputer configuration) used to process research tapes when accurate counts of PVC incidence are required. The ARGUS system was developed at Washington University (5) in St. Louis and adapted to the needs of the Thoraxcentre (6). Firstly, digitization is performed at 120 times real-time, followed by the actual analysis which is automatic. There is then a machine edit phase requiring some operator intervention. This is followed by all beats labeled PVC by the computer system being presented to the operator for review. The last step is a quality control edit where the operator reviews all the data in a 30 minute segment selected from the full 24-hour tape.

The selection criteria for the quality control block, are that the data must be of reasonable quality (≤30% bad data) and that the block with the highest percentage of early, non-PVC beats is to be selected. The reason for this selection is two-fold. Firstly it is most likely to contain the largest number of missed PVCs and at the same time it enables registration of a count of the number of supra-ventricular premature beats, which are not counted by the ARGUS system. The overhead of this quality control edit is not very high on average. Figure 4 shows

12

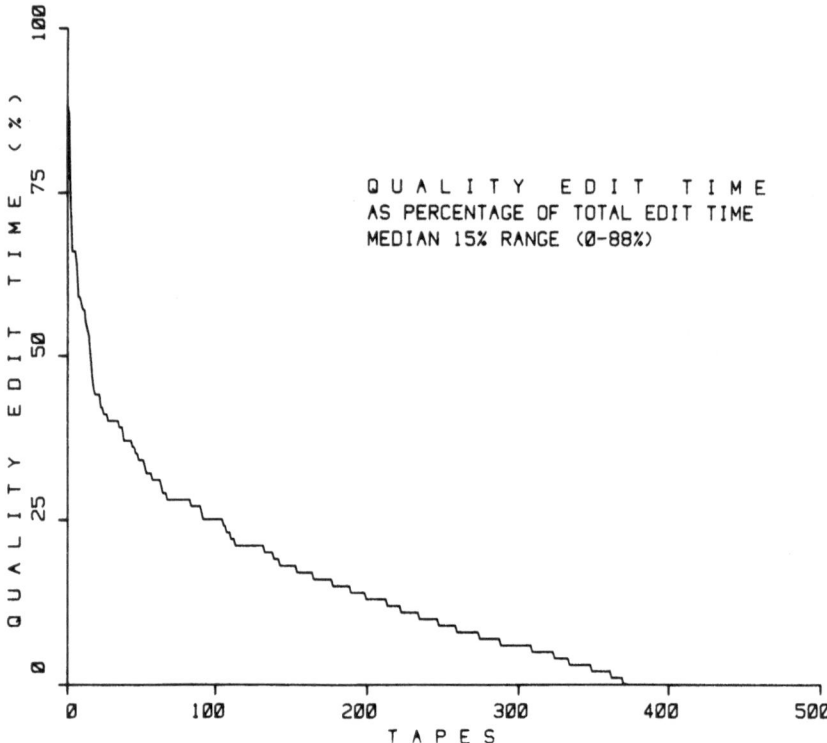

Figure 5. Quality Control Editing Time.

the distribution of the editing time for 380 sequentially processed tapes, it varied between 15 minutes and 22 hours with a median value of 37 minutes, while figure 5 indicates the cost of the quality control procedure in terms of operator time, a median of 15% of total operator time per tape was spent on the quality control procedure.

Figure 6 shows the number of isolated PVCs found in each of 500 tapes during the standard edit and during the quality control procedure. As might be expected, there were virtually no false positive PVCs (only 13 in a total of approximately 1.000.000 beats analysed), since they had been eliminated in the normal editing process. On the other hand, only 88% of all PVCs had been detected by the computer. This is probably an underestimate of the overall performance, however, since the quality control block was selected to yield a potentially high percentage of false negatives.

In the 500 quality control blocks, a total of 137 couplets were found, 94% of these were correctly detected by the ARGUS system, while no false-positives occurred. Only one of the 500 quality control blocks showed runs of more than 2 PVCs. 41 out of 45 of these runs had been correctly detected by the system.

This type of quality control is a self-reference in that the operator acts as 'gold standard'. A refinement is to have tapes scanned by another operator, perhaps

	QUALITY CONTROL				
	0	1	2	3	≥4
0	285	13			3
1		50	4		3
2	1		19	1	1
3	1			10	7
≥4					102

Figure 6. Number of Isolated PVC's in 500 30 Minute Segments.

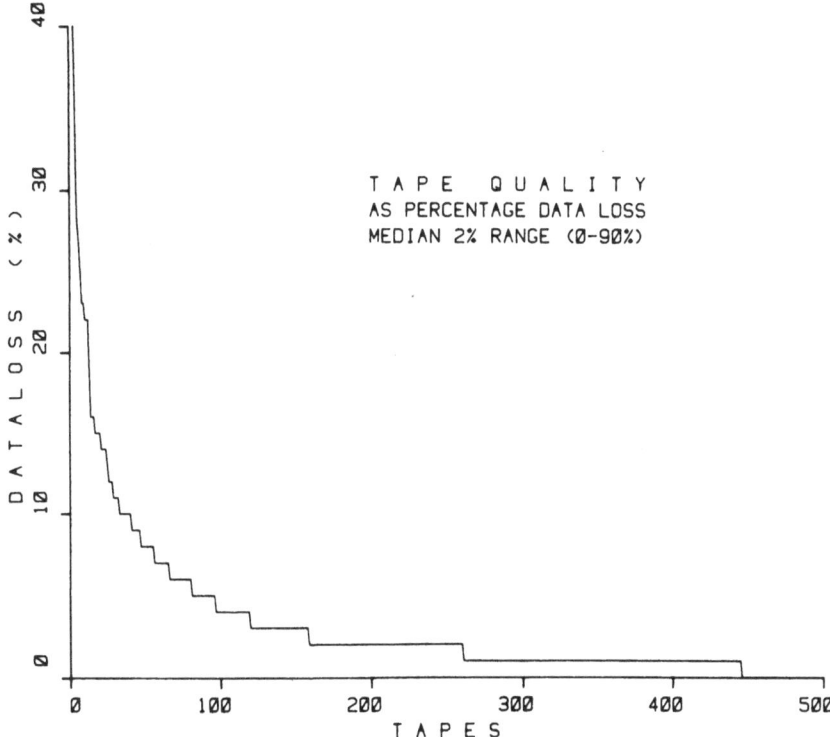

Figure 7. Tape Quality Overall Results.

14

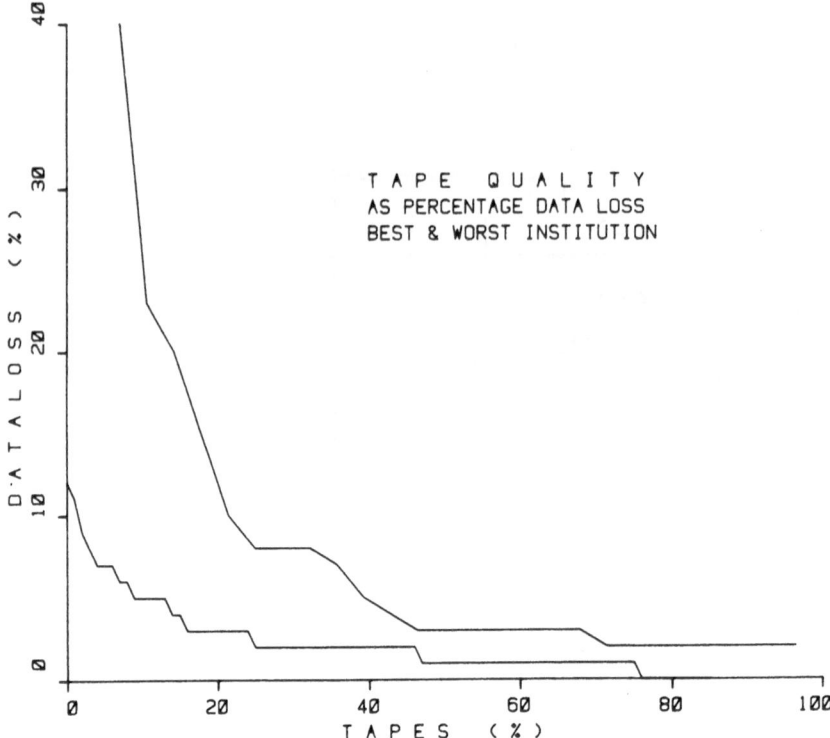

Figure 8. Tape Quality per Institution.

on a random sample basis, since questions of expense will normally preclude much double reading. Application of this type of quality control to small, randomly selected segments of tape can also be combined with fully automated scanning (once system characteristics are well understood) in order to provide a facility with a higher capacity than the average, research-oriented, system employing operator editing. Such a facility is appropriate, for instance, for the evaluation of therapy where extreme accuracy in ventricular arrhythmia counting is unnecessary but overall accuracy is essential, since the system report can relate directly to the therapeutic intervention performed.

Another aspect of quality control concerns the signal quality of the tapes analysed. Figure 7 shows the tape quality expressed as the percentage of total data that could be analysed by the computer system. This is of course only an approximation of what is subjectively seen as 'tape quality' but at least it provides a level of quantitation. The median and mean data loss was here only 2%, but, as figure 8 shows, results varied widely over different institutions. The quality control procedure can, in this case, be used directly as a feedback to participating institutions in order to improve tape quality and, as a direct consequence, analysis results.

In conclusion, a clear specification of system functions and user requirements is essential when selecting equipment for Holter tape analysis. This must be clearly matched to the system specification put forward by the supplier and care taken to ensure that the 'fancy' (and often unnecessary) aspects of the design do not obscure the essential qualities, good or bad, of the equipment. Performance measures of Holter analysis equipment are important for both manufacturers and buyers of these systems. They provide an objective means of comparison and evaluation. Annotated arrhythmia databases will hopefully provide an important tool to make this kind of assessment possible for at least the class of ventricular arrhythmia detectors. Quality control is essential for service providers and customers alike. A well-defined procedure with a clear protocol helps both to promote the users' trust in the system and to reveal weak spots in the analysis process. It can be carried out for a relatively low percentage of total analysis cost.

References

1. Computers in Cardiology, Bethesda, Maryland. IEEE Computer Society, Long Beach California, No. 74CHO879–7C, pp. 21–27.
.2. Hermes RE, Geselowitz DB, Oliver GCh. 1980. Development, distribution, and use of the American Heart Association database for ventricular arrhythmia detector evaluation. Computers in Cardiology, Williamsburg, Virginia. IEEE Computer Society, Long Beach California, No. 80CH1606–3, pp. 262–266.
3. Schluter P, Mark R, Moody G, Olson W, Peterson S. 1980. Performance measures for arrhythmia detectors. Computers in Cardiology, Williamsburg, Virginia. IEEE Computer Society, Long Beach California, No. 80CH1606–3, pp. 267–270.
4. Hermes RE, Cox, Jr. JR. 1980. A methodology for performance evaluation of ventricular arrhythmia detectors. Computers in Cardiology, Williamsburg, Virginia. IEEE Computer Society, Long Beach California, No. 80CH1606–3, pp. 3–8.
5. Clark KW, Hitschens RE, Ritter JA, Rankin SL, Oliver GC, Thomas, Jr. LJ. 1977. Argus/2H: a dual-channel holter-tape analysis system. Computers in Cardiology, Rotterdam, The Netherlands. IEEE Computer Society, Long Beach California, No. 77CH1254–2C, pp. 191–198.
6. Ripley KL, Okkerse, RJ, Engelse WAH, Vinke RVH, Zeelenberg C. 1980. Implementation of Argus/2H at the Thoraxcentrum. Computers in Cardiology, Williamsburg, Virginia. IEEE Computer Society, Long Beach California, No. 80CH1606–3, pp. 135–138.

CLINICAL IMPORTANCE OF COMPUTER ASSISTED
LONG-TERM ECG ANALYSIS

H.S. WEBER, G. JOSKOWICZ, D. GLOGAR, K.K. STEINBACH, F. KAINDL

1. Introduction

Since 1961 the present golden standard in the noninvasive investigations of arrhythmias is the Holter technique (1). The main advantages of storing 24 hours ECG continuously under ambulatory conditions on magnetic tapes are the local independence, the relatively constant signal quality, the simple handling of the recording units and the poor influence of this method on patient's way of life. Technical problems occur when the stored ECG has to be evaluated as fast and as reliable as possible. Thus most of the effort has been spent in the development of fast and efficient playback- and analysis units.

2. Analysis Methods

The most simple analysis method is the *audio-visual screening* of the high-speed played back record. During the last years this method was supplemented by the application of UV-printers, which could write out the ECG on-line from the playback unit despite the high frequency content of the signal. The results are ECG-strips, which need a time-consuming further interpretation process by a well-trained physician. Today in daily routine *hardware oriented systems* are commonly used because of their high throughput, their off-the-shelf availability and their amount of clinical important informations.

Computer assisted analysis including special signal conditioning algorithms opened a new field of highly reliable informations especially with regard to the context of heart rhythm, arrhythmias, symptoms and cardiac death.

The *"social acceptable monitoring instruments"* (SAMI) represent a new class of synchronous recording/analysis systems emerging from the development of semiconductor technology and of solid state memories. Only small parts of the ECG curve or some descriptors like heart rate can be stored because of limited capacity of that memories today. The advantages of this method are the extended recording time over days and weeks without restrictions of patient's life and the

SOFTWARE AND HARDWARE BASED SYSTEMS
IN LONG TERM-ECG ANALYSIS

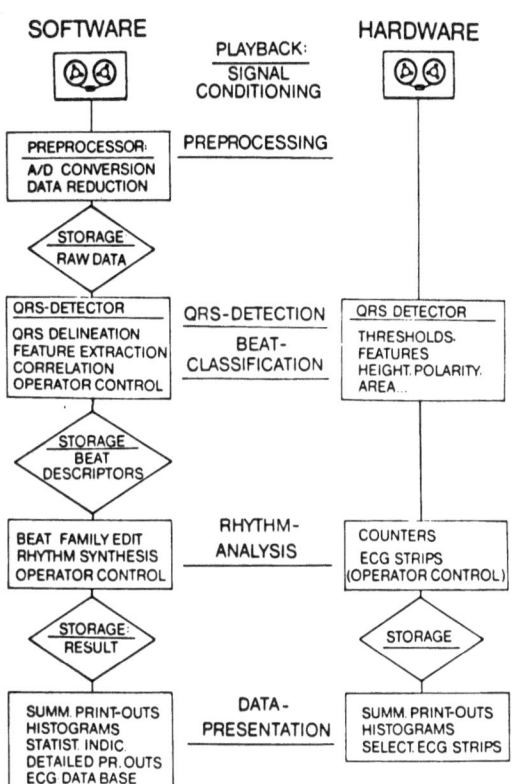

Figure 1.

neglegible playback and read out time. Different realisations of such instruments are possible, but common to all is the fact that it remains impossible to recover the primary information out of such a "black box".

Therefore at present we have to deal with hardware oriented and computer supported systems.

3. Software and Hardware Based Systems

Due to the fast development of microelectronics the difference between software oriented systems and normal scanners is not easy to describe. The main characteristics of software oriented computer supported systems, which have been proposed till now (2, 3, 4, 5), are the preprocessing of the ECG signal including A/D-conversion, data reduction (fig. 1) and the use of large random access disks (5–160 MB). They allow the algorithm to make use of more contextual informations.

Hardware oriented systems (fig. 1), which use also microprocessors today, can only access data in a sequential way. This limits the possibilities of the algorithms in use. Whereas software oriented systems can store intermediary results together with the raw data (fig. 2), e.g. the beat descriptor file. This allows the use of very sophisticated editing algorithms under continuous operator control and computer-operator communication with interactive intervention.

In computer assisted systems artefact detecting algorithms reduce the number of false positive results due to signal noise, baselinedrift and muscle artefacts in contrast to hardware oriented systems. In our system (5) we use e.g. a multistage artefact detection: During data acquisition a noisy signal will be detected when the signal to noise ratio overestimates an adjustable value. Those parts of the ECG will be skipped. During QRS-delineation deflections which do not fit into QRS-descriptors are also considered as artefacts (fig. 2). And at last during the automated QRS-editing process (fig. 1): extremely shortened or prolonged RR-intervals will be presented automatically on display for operator's decision.

Data presentation (fig. 1) of independent results enhances the redundancy of detected arrhythmias in computer supported analysis. That means that the number of e.g. normal beats or PVCs occur once in the summarized print-out and second in a numerical RR- and/or QRS-area-histogram. Both results are achieved during different analysis processes so that identical data demonstrate the result's plausibility. On the other hand hardware oriented systems can only use stop-and-go operations to check their reliability.

The intermediate data storage allows also more sophisticated sorting which is used in the computation of statistical indicators, e.g. dependence of the PVC frequency from the heart rate. Commonly software oriented systems are used for research and seem to be moretime consuming than hardware oriented systems.

4. Time Consumption in Software and Hardware Oriented Systems

One important question in long-term ECG analysis is the time requirement to achieve results of comparable high quality using different systems. We analysed 12 randomly selected tapes with different QRS features, signal quality and tape content routinely with the available computer assisted system and with two commercial hardware oriented systems.

4.1. Computer Supported "Multipass Scanning" (Fig. 1)

It is based on well known approaches (3, 5). After A/D-conversion and data-reduction using the "Linear Segmentation Technique"(5) in a 4 x 4 bit slice micro-processor the raw data are stored on 5 MB disks. The analysis is performed in two passes. During the first pass the QRS detector and delineator groups similar QRS-complexes into feature clusters. During the second pass the primitives of the beat families are synthesized to complex rhythm diagnoses under operator control and interactions. Characteristic examples of complex arrhythmias are stored on a data base and can be resynthesized from the digitized data and strip charted. Such strategies were presuppositions for the high reliability of that system evaluated by visual beat-to-beat scanning: The QRS detector demonstrated a specificity of 97,7% and a sensitivity of 99,7% over 77.000 heart beats. Analog data for PVC delineation over 1700 multiform PVCs were 99,8% specificity and 96,5% sensitivity (6).

4.2. Hardware Oriented Systems

Reynold's "Pathfinder" (7) and Hittman's "Compu-Scan" analyse the ECG directly from the high speed playback (fig. 1). The latter one can reach a maximal speed of 240 x recording speed dependant from the heart rate. The "Pathfinder" (PF) features a variety of manual controls for setting up the QRS-discriminator. The possibilities in "Compu-Scan" (CS) are restricted on the QRS-area difference and on the prematurity. As mentioned above, stop-and-go operations must be included in both systems to check the result's reliability; in PF only during the analysis. Both systems have provisions for numerical trend print-outs and graphic displays for data presentation.

4.3. Tape Quality and Content

The 12 tapes selected from daily routine demonstrated in 60% (7 tapes over 146 hrs) a high signal quality with a mean artefact rate of <5%. In two tapes (over 43 hrs) the artefact rates were between 5 and 10% and in the remaining three tapes (63 hrs) the signal quality was poor (artefact rate >10%). In 8 tapes (75%) normal sinus-rhythm without significant ventricular arrhythmias predominated, 5 with high signal quality and 2 with high artefact rates. In the remaining 4 tapes over 81 hrs a mean PVC-rate of >5% and/or complex ventricular arrhythmias occurred.

4.4. Duration of Analysis

The *preanalysis time*, e.g. the time before the ECG analysis itself can start, consisted of the playback time of max. 24 min. in "Multipass-Scanning" (MP-SC). Both hardware oriented systems needed less than 10 min. to set up the system.

The mean *analysis time* differed much between the used systems; Operator interactions and semiautomatic pre- and rechecking of the disk-stored data led to a mean analysis duration of 56 ± 36 min. in MP-SC. In the PF system a mean analysis time of 24 ± 4 min. occurred, whereas the high speed play back in CS led to a demand of 10 ± 3 min. for analysis.

To recheck the quality of the obtained results a *correction pass* using the "roll-and-jogg" technique was necessary in CS, which needed mean 54 ± 51 min. MP-SC never needed such a correction pass because of their continuous, operator observed quality control during the whole analysis (8). In PF further correction steps were impossible, because that system has no provisions to retrieve specific events.

The *total analysis time* (TAT) in MP-SC consisted only of the analysis time of 56 ± 36 min. neglecting the preanalysis time in a multiprocessing environment. In CS the TAT exceeded with 65 ± 52 min. the TAT of the software oriented system, whereas the time consumption in the PF system was only 28 ± 8 min. disregarding the impossibility to recheck the quality of the analysis.

The mean *TAT per recorded hour* (MP-SC: 2,7 ± 2 min., PF: 1,4 ± 0,4 min., CS: 3,3 ± 3 min.) was independant from the tape quality in MP-SC, but clearly positive correlated in both hardware oriented systems (PF: r=0,531, p<0,05; CS: r=0,848, p<0,001). The computer assisted system (MP-SC) detects artefacts like signal noise, baseline drift, etc. correctly and eliminates such ECG segments. In hardware oriented systems (PF, CS) such artefacts increase the number of false positive detected heart beats and PVCs and should need further correction steps despite signal-noice detectors. The tape content increased the TAT/HR in MP-SC (tab. 1) because of a higher amount of annotated phenomena on display for operator's manual decision. In CS the further correction pass enhances also the TAT/HR in relation to the tape content (tab. 1). It seems to be obvious that the constant TAT/HR in PF is influenzed by the amount of stop-and-go operations and of number of ECG strips written out during the analysis. If such operations will be initiated more frequently in complex arrhythmias the time consumption will increase too. The small number of complex ventricular arrhythmias and strip-charted ECGs feign a TAT/HR-independency from the tape content (tab. 1).

TAPE CONTENT AND TAT/HR

TAT/HR (MIN)

	$\leq$	A	B
MP-SC	2,7 ± 2	1,9 ± 0,7	4,4 ± 2,3
PF	1,4 ± 0,4	1,4 ± 0,4	1,4 ± 0,4
CS	3,3 ± 3	3,0 ± 3,7	4,2 ± 2,0

Table 1: Leg.: TAT/HR: Total analysis time of one hour recorded ECG. A: Tapes with different signal quality, but predominantly normal sinus-rhythm. B: Tapes with different signal quality, but with a mean PVC rate of > 5% and/or complex ventricular arrhythmias. MP-SC: Computer assisted "Multipass-Scanning" analysis system. PF and CS: hardware oriented analysis systems "Pathfinder" and "Compu-Scan".

4.5. Summary:

— Software oriented systems are more time consuming than hardware oriented systems.
— Hardware oriented systems need a further correction pass to achieve as reliable results as software oriented systems.
— So the total analysis time demonstrates no large difference between both methods if a result of high quality is needed.
— The analysis time in software oriented systems is independent from the tape quality and from the artefact rate,
— but is directly correlated to the tape content similar to hardware systems: Increasing amount of complex arrhythmias leads to an increasing amount either of operator interactions or of stop-and-go operations (ECG strips) or correction steps following the analysis.

5. Main Indications for Longterm ECG

Four main indications lead to an increasing demand for the Holter investigation in the clinical routine:
— Symptoms possibly caused by arrhythmias;
— general questions for present arrhythmias and their characteristics;
— evaluation of antiarrhythmic therapy and
— pacemaker control.

5.1. Symptomatic Patients

Symptoms like dizzy spells, syncopes, palpitations, paroxysmal tachycardias and pulse irregularities can be based on arrhythmias. To capture such a symptomatic period with a 24 hrs Holter monitoring a typical event must occur minimal once a day disregarding its duration. Out of 53 patients 51% developed such a symptomatic event during one 24 hrs longterm ECG, whereas in 30% arrhythmias could be excluded as reason for the symptoms (9). If the symptoms occur less frequent than once within 24 hrs either repetitive longterm ECGs or patient initiated or automatic event recorders (10) or ECG-telephone-transmission can be used. To register the ECG during a symptomatic period in 50% of 100 patients with syncopes in their history. Johansson (11) needed a mean continuous recording duration over 4 days (1–22 days). Patient initiated event recorders lead only to some ECG strips. The ECG telephone transmission is especially limited through the duration of the symptomatic period. Symptoms have to last until a successfully telephone connection with the recording center is obtained (12). Both methods, Holter monitoring and ECG telephone transmission led to success in 60% of the patients (9), whereas in 1/3, arrhythmias as reason for the symptoms could be excluded and in the remaining 1/3 confirmed (9). In all this above mentioned methods computer assisted and/or hardware oriented analysis of long-term ECG records are either unnecessary or of limited value. ECG strips of the symptomatic period will lead to satisfactory diagnoses with less time consumption and costs.

5.2. Recognition of Arrhythmias

The suspicion for arrhythmias, commonly asymptomatic, and 12-lead-ECG-recorded arrhythmias are the domain of semiautomatic hardware or software oriented analysis including qualification and quantification of the actual rhythm. The application of computer assisted analysis was followed by an increasing amount of new informations about the heart rhythm and its disturbances. Doubts appeared in the common used concepts of arrhythmias interpretation and therapeutic strategies.

5.3. Evaluation of Antiarrhythmic Therapy

The second domain of semiautomatic analysis is the quantitative and qualitative evaluation of antiarrhythmic therapy. Circadian and spontaneous variabilities of arrhythmias (13, 14) uncover the problematic of "successful" antiarrhythmic treatment: Such mentioned phenomena can mimick a therapeutic success (15). Therefore infrequent arrhythmias, under or without therapy demonstrating a high variability need a prolongation of the monitoring duration to overcome such spontaneous and circadian variabilities:

F (frequency) X L (monitoring duration) = V (variability)

Nevertheless longterm ECG and its different analysis methods are the most valuable tools to answer the question how to treat arrhythmias in the future.

5.4. Pacemaker Control:

In principle longterm ECG is not the method of choice for PM control. But often PM malfunction (exit block, sensing defects etc.) are infrequent phenomena, occurring sudden and unexpected during daily life. So 24 hrs continuous ECG registration under ambulatory conditions will be able to capture such rare events. The registration of the PM-spike is simple. But using high speed play back the frequency content of the spikes increases so much that new detection methods had to be developed to recognize the spike with high accuracy. The spike will be stored on a separate track of the magnetic tape. Prior A/D-conversion the spike will be lengthened so that similar to the event marker the now rectangular impulse can be recognized despite the high playback speed. The detection of a PM-spike initiates in MP-SC the PM-logic that relates PM-spikes with the previous and subsequent QRS complexes. Such developed devices for VVI (16) and for AAI-PM (17) were only used for research programs. A very recent report (18) describes a combined hardware ("Pathfinder") and software oriented analysis method using a preprocessor for PM-spike detection. The first clinical data seems to be very fruitful in the detection of PM-malfunctions. By now the analysis of longterm PM-recordings (computer assisted, hardware oriented or both) is far away from use in the clinical routine. But the demand of such a kind of PM supervision under ambulatory conditions increases with the introduction of microprocessors in todays PM-technology − from the clinical point of view.

5.5. Summary

− In symptomatic patients semiautomatic analysis methods of Holter monitoring are not the method of choice.
− The main indications for both analysis methods, computer assisted versus hardware oriented, are the recognition, quantification and qualification of suspected or present arrhythmias.
− Another domain is the control of antiarrhythmic therapy without neglection of arrhythmia's variabilities.
− Modern PM technology will increase the demand of PM analysis systems in the nearest future.

6. Physician's Demand

In our Holter center, when calling for a longterm ECG investigation, the physician has to describe his expectations on an admission form. This is because from a methodological point of view, one can only recognize an object which is anticipated. Furthermore a questionnaire is attached to each report leaving the laboratory. It consists of two sets of questions, which have to be answered by the assigning physician: Does the report meet the expectations? What consequences can be derived from that report? Thus a very close feedback mechanism was established with the computer assisted longterm ECG analysis system in the clinical routine.

6.1. User's Expectations

The suspicion of present arrhythmias led in 49% of the patients to the longterm ECG investigation (fig. 2). Reasons for that suspicions were symptoms possibly related to arrhythmias, as mentioned above in 28%. In the remaining 21% the physicians needed more detailed informations about rare occurring but just

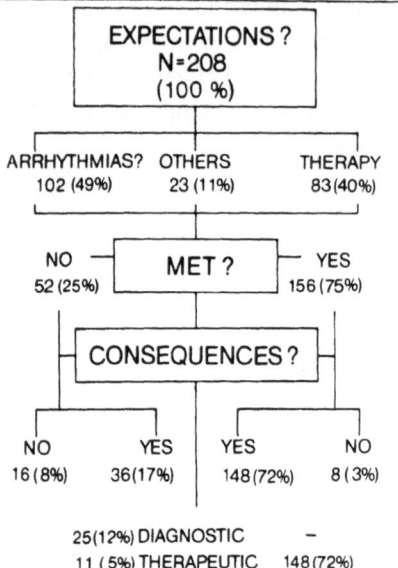

COMPUTER ASSISTED
LONG TERM-ECG ANALYSIS:

EVALUATION USING A QUESTIONNAIRE

EXPECTATIONS ?
N=208
(100 %)

ARRHYTHMIAS?   OTHERS   THERAPY
102 (49%)   23 (11%)   83 (40%)

NO   MET ?   YES
52 (25%)   156 (75%)

CONSEQUENCES ?

NO   YES   YES   NO
16 (8%) 36(17%) 148(72%)   8 (3%)

25(12%) DIAGNOSTIC   —
11 (5%) THERAPEUTIC   148(72%)

Figure 2.

documented arrhythmias.

The second major indication for Holter monitoring was the evaluation and control of antiarrhythmic therapy in 40%. In the remaining 11% questions for PM-indication, PM-malfunctions, individual rhythm behaviour during stress etc. had to be answered.

6.2. Questionnaire

Answered questionnaires were only used in patients investigated routinely and excluded from research programs. From 336 questionnaires 62% were returned.

6.2.1. Expectations   Met. The above mentioned expectations were met in 156 out of 208 patients (fig. 2).

In the remaining 52 pts Holter monitoring failed because of too short recording time (24 hrs) to capture suspected events (12%), or because of technical problems (9%): Hardware failure (5%), poor signal quality (4%), so that no reliable result could be obtained. In 4% no informations came back, why the Holter investigation

6.2.2. Met Expectations and Consequences (N=156 pts). The met expectations led in 115 pts (56%) to therapeutic consequences (fig. 2), commonly pharmacological therapy (53,5%): In 27 pts the report was followed by initiation of antiarrhythmic therapy, in 14% (30 pts) followed by changing the used drugs. In 49% the drug regimen was successful, so that the physician decided to continue. In 5 pts the physician stopped unnecessary medications (fig. 2).

Surgical interventions were PM-implantation in 3 pts and in one pat. aneurysmectomy.

No therapeutic management was necessary in 33 pts (16%). No consequences were derived despite a conclusive report in 8 pts (3%).

6.2.3. Disappointed Expectations and Consequences (N=52 pts). If the report did not fulfill the user's expectations further diagnostic steps were necessary in 12% (25 pts): In 14 pts Holter monitoring was repeated. The monitoring duration over 24 hrs continuously seemed to be too short to capture rare but suspected phenomena or symptoms. In 5% disappointing results led to further cardiologic investigations (9 pts noninvasive, one patient each electrophysiologic testing and heart catheterization). Despite an inconclusive report in 5% therapeutic consequences followed: 2 pts underwent PM-implantation. In 5 pts actual drug regimen was continued.

Failing long-term ECG and no further diagnostic or therapeutic consequences were reported in 16 pts (8%). The lack of feedback informations led to an obviously "overinvestigation" in those pts, in whom other diagnostic tools seemed to be necessary for full success.

6.3. Kind of Data for Report's Conclusion

6.3.1. Data Representation. Data presentation in longterm ECG consists of:
— the *summarized data* of detected heart beats, PVCs etc. (SPO),
— of *histograms* which show up time correlated trends, and of *statistical indicators* (STI) correlating measured parameters (e.g. PVC frequency with actual heart rate).
— The *detailed printout* (DPO) and *ECG strips* represent the individual description of clinical relevant phenomena either in numerical form or in strip charted ECGs, directly from the magnetic tape during stop-and-go-operations (hardware oriented systems), or resynthesized from digitized data stored in a data base (computer assisted analysis, MP-SC).

6.3.2. Kind of Data Meeting the Expectations (N=156 pts). In 26,5% of the reports with met expectations only either SPO (7%), STI (3%) or DPO (26,5%) were necessary to obtain the conclusive result (fig. 3). In 51,5% (80 pts) a combination of two different types of data presentation and in 12% (19 pts) all three had to be applied to return the expected informations. The summarized printout alone

KIND OF DATA FOR REPORT'S CONCLUSIONS

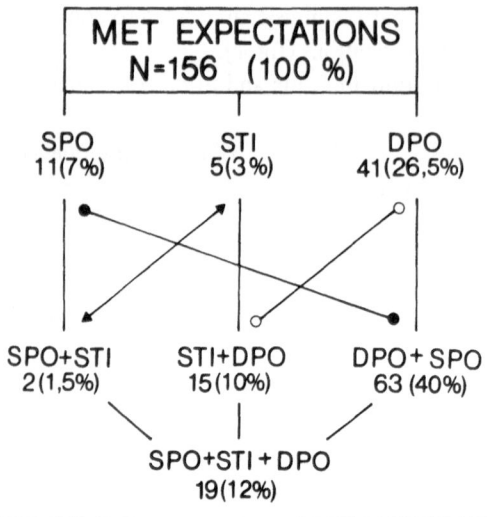

MET EXPECTATIONS
N=156 (100 %)

SPO 11(7%) STI 5(3%) DPO 41(26,5%)

SPO+STI 2(1,5%) STI+DPO 15(10%) DPO+SPO 63 (40%)

SPO+STI+DPO 19(12%)

SPO SUMMARIZED PRINTOUT
DPO DETAILED PRINTOUT
STI STATISTICAL INDICATORS

Figure 3.

or combined with the other types was of value in 95 of the reports (60,5%). Histograms and/or statistical indicators influenced the result only in 26% (41 pts), because of absent numerical and quantitative description of data in histogram form. Today the value of statistical indicators is underestimated, but their value will increase, when clinical important informations for therapeutic strategies can be derived. A detailed description of clinical relevant arrhythmias, exact time correlated, was the most valuable part of data presentation in longterm ECG analysis. The detailed printout was essential for conclusive reports in 88,5% (135 pts).

6.4. Summary:

— Physician's expectations are the question for arrhythmias present and for the evaluation of antiarrhythmic therapy, when they call for Holter monitoring.
— The expectations can be fulfilled in 75%.
— Met expectations lead to therapeutic consequences in 72%.
— A detailed description of clinical important arrhythmias (numerical form or strip charted ECG) was necessary in 88,5% of the conclusive reports.

7. Conclusions

7.1. Computer assisted long-term ECG analysis is more time consuming compared to software oriented systems, especially if screening predominantly tapes of highest signal quality and normal tape content.

7.2. If artefact rate and/or tape content increase the analysistime approximates particularly if reliable results should be obtained.

7.3. The time consuming parts in discriminator analysis are the performance of detailed data using stop-and-go-operations with or without strip charted ECGs.

7.4. To fulfill the expectations of the physicians in the clinical routine in 75% of the requested reports detailed data presentation will be needed in 88,5% of the conclusive reports.

7.5. So computer assisted long-term-ECG analysis with highly reliable and redundant data, achieved under continuous operator control, cannot be used only for research, but also successfully and economically in the clinical routine.

Acknowledgement

We are indebted to thank Mrs. U. Groyer, A. Reich and T. Haagen for their technical assistance.

References

1. Holter, N.J. 1961: New method for heart studies. Science 134, 1214 ff.
2. Spitz, A.L., Harrison, D.C. 1978: Automated family classification in ambulatory monitoring. Med. Instr. p. 225.
3. Mead, C.N., Clark, K.W., Potter, S.T., Moore, S.M., Thomas, L.J. Jr. 1979: Development and evaluation of a new QRS detector/delineator. Comp. Card. (IEEE) p. 251−254.
4. Birman, K.P., Rolnitzky, L.M., Bigger, J.T. Jr. 1978: A shape oriented system for automated Holter ECG analysis. Comp. Card. (IEEE) p. 217 ff.
5. Joskowicz, G., Balatka, H., Glogar, D., Weber, H., Steinbach, K. 1978: A high speed digital Holter tape analysis with ful editing capability. 1979 Comp. Card. (IEEE) p. 277−280.
6. Weber, H., Joskowicz, G., Glogar, D., Steinbach, K., Probst, P., Kaindl, F. 1981. Proceedings of ISAM, in Press.
7. Neilson, J.M. 1974: High speed analysis of ventricular arrhythmias from 24 hrs recordings. Comp. Card. (IEEE) p. 55−61.
8. Weber, H., Glogar, D., Joskowicz, G., Steinbach, K., Kaindl, F. 1978: Continuous and systematic quality control in ambulatory ECG. In E. Sandøe, D.G. Julian, J.W. Bell: Management of ventricular tachycardia-role of Mexiletine, p. 358 ff.
9. Scheibelhofer, W., Weber, H.S., Joskowicz, G., Glogar, D., Probst, P., Steinbach, K.,

Kaindl, K. 1981: Symptom correlated ECG-registration using longterm ECG and ECG telephone telemetry. In ISAM, Gent, in Press.

10. Mark, R.G., Moody, G.B., Olson, W.H., Peterson, S.K. 1980: Event recorders and future systems. In N. Kass-Wnger, M.B. Mock, I. Rinquist: Ambulatory electrocardiographic recording, p. 113–132.

11. Abdow, N.J., Lecerof, H., Johansson, D.E. 1980: Electrophysiological examination or monitoring in suspected Adams-Stokes-Syndrome? Pace 2, p. 94 ff.

12. Weber, H., Steinbach, K., Joskowicz, G., Glogar, D., Kaindl, F. 1980: TTM versus Holter monitoring of symptomatic arrhythmias. Am. Heart J. 100, p. 764–765.

13. Morganroth, J.E., Michelson, E.L., Hornath, L.N., Josephson, M.E., Pearlman, A.S., Dunkman, W.B. 1978: Limitations of routine longterm ambulatory electrocardiographic monitoring to assess ventricular ectopic frequency. Circulation 58, p. 408 .

14. Lown, D., Tykocinski, M., Garfen, A., Brooks, Ph. 1973: Sleep and ventricular premature beats. Circulation 48, p. 691.

15. Winkle, R.A. 1978: Antiarrhythmic drug effect mimicked by spontaneous variability of ventricular ectopy. Circulation 57, 1116.

16. Steinbach, K., Glogar, D., Huber, J., Joskowicz, G., Weber, H. 1978: Longterm Monitoring for detection of failure of the pacemaker/ electrode system and arrhythmias. 1st. Europ. Symposion on Cardiac Pacing. The Pacemaker Follow up. p. 53–54.

17. Weber, H., Glogar, D., Joskowicz, G., Steinbach K., Probst, P., Kaindl, F., Laczkovics, A. 1981: Computer assisted longterm ECG analysis in patients with artificial atrial pacemaker (AAI) Z. f. Kardiol. 70, 151–157.

18. Murray, A., Jordan, R.S. 1981: Analysis of ECG recordings from pacemaker patients. Comp. Card. (IEEE), Florenz, in Press.

HOLTER MONITORING IN THE EVALUATION OF PALPITATIONS, DIZZINESS AND SYNCOPE

D. BURCKHARDT, B.E. LUETOLD, M.V. JOST, A. HOFFMANN

1. Introduction

Long-term ambulatory electrocardiographic (Holter) monitoring is widely used to evaluate patients presenting with palpitations, dizziness and syncope (1). Most of the reports in the literature show a high prevalence of arrhythmias in patients studied for these indications and conclude that the method is very useful (2–5). However, a strong link between symptoms and arrhythmias has only been shown in a small proportion of cases (6, 7) and the value of the method must be weighed against its costs (7).

The purpose of the present study was to assess the yield of Holter-monitoring in the evaluation of patients with palpitations, dizziness and syncope and to establish the prevalence of arrhythmias and their correlation with symptoms. A further aim of the study was to assess Holter findings in a subgroup of patients who continued to complain of syncope or dizziness despite the implantation of a pacemaker for documented brady-arrhythmias.

2. Material and Methods

2.1. Procedure

From September 1979 through March 1981 a total of 950 Holter tracings were recorded by our department. 165 (17,4%) of these were performed because of palpitations and 240 (25,2%) were requested for the evaluation of dizziness and syncope. The remainder of all tracings were done to assess antiarrhythmic drug efficacy and for detection of arrhythmias in groups of asymptomatic patients with heart disease (Fig. 1).

All tapes were recorded on a Dynagram model 5000 cassette recorder with the exploring electrode in V_5 position. The cassettes were replayed at 60 times real speed on a model 6004 C Holter cardiography system* and printed beat on

---

* Instruments for Cardiac Research Corporation, Syracuse, New York, USA.

Long-term ambulatory
electrocardiography   FdB

Reasons for Holter Monitoring

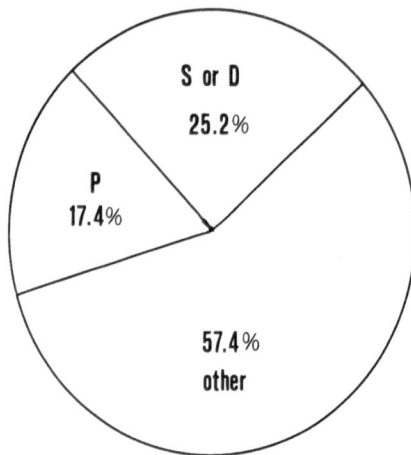

S or D = Syncope or Dizziness
P = Palpitations
N = 950

Figure 1. Reasons for Holter monitoring in 950 patients.

beat on fiberoptic paper**. Detailed real time printouts of relevant strips were available. The material was then analyzed manually by a trained cardiologist. Patients were instructed to keep an exact record of their usual daily activities and of symptoms. A symptom was accepted as correlating with an arrhythmia if they occurred within 5 minutes of one another. Palpitations were defined as skipped beats, irregular or rapid heart action or increased awareness of heart action.

2.2. Definitions

ST   = sinus tachycardia = 100 beats/min.
SVEA = supraventricular ectopic activity, including:
    APB's : frequent atrial premature beats (>30 per hour)
    SVT   : paroxysmal supraventricular tachycardia (=10 consecutive beats with abrupt onset and with a heart rate of = 130/min.)
    AF   : intermittent atrial flutter or fibrillation
VEA   = ventricular ectopic activity of Lown grade II-V (8).
Major tachy-arrhythmias: supraventricular tachycardia, atrial flutter, atrial fibrillation, couplets of VPBs or VT (= 3 VPBs in a row).

** Honeywell Visicorder 1856 A.

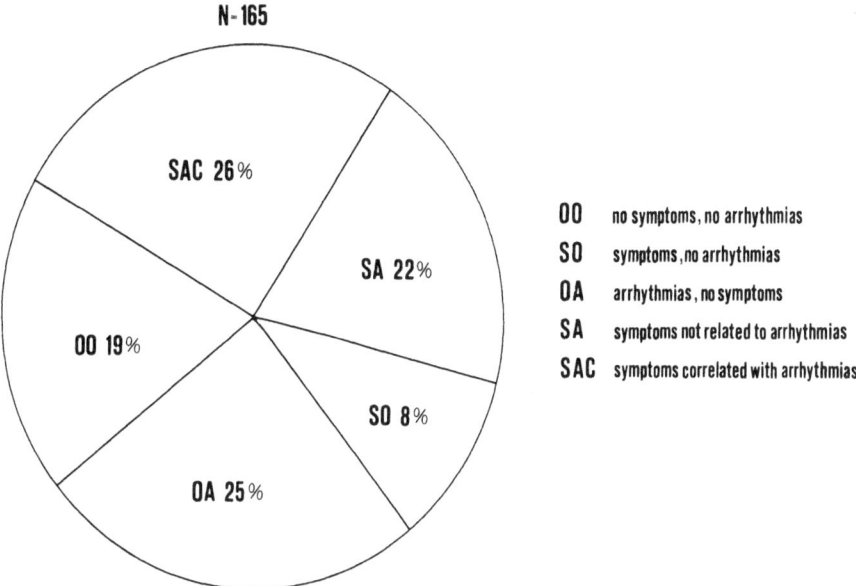

N-165

SAC 26%

SA 22%

OO 19%

SO 8%

OA 25%

OO   no symptoms, no arrhythmias
SO   symptoms, no arrhythmias
OA   arrhythmias, no symptoms
SA   symptoms not related to arrhythmias
SAC symptoms correlated with arrhythmias

Figure 2. Findings on Holter tracings in 165 patients evaluated for palpitations.

Major brady-arrhythmias: sinus bradycardia of <40/min, second degree AV block or third degree AV block, SA block, sinus arrest of more than 2 seconds.

3. Results

3.1. Evaluation of Palpitations

3.1.1. Characteristics of Patients. 165 patients (84 men, 81 women) were evaluated for palpitations. Their age ranged from 18–83 years (mean 54). The mean duration of ECG recording was 23 hours (range 5–48), and was at least 24 hours in 81% of studies.

Ninety-two of these patients (56%) experienced palpitations during monitoring. In 120 of 165 patients (73%) an arrhythmia (ST, VEA, AF or a combination of these) was observed (Fig. 2). Thirteen patients (8%) experienced symptoms without showing arrhythmias. In 36 patients (22%) both symptoms and arrhythmias occurred during monitoring but these were not related to each other. A correlation of symptoms and arrhythmias was observed in 43 patients (26% of all patients or 47% of symptomatic studies).

3.1.2. Prevalence of Arrhythmias in Patients Evaluated for Palpitations. In 45 of the 165 patients (27%), no arrhythmias were observed. Eighteen (11%) showed ST, 32 (20%) SVEA, 48 (30%) VEA and 20 (12%) combined SVEA + VEA. In supraventricular arrhythmias, frequent APB's, SVT and AF were equally distributed (Fig. 3).

ARRHYTHMIAS IN PATIENTS WITH PALPITATIONS

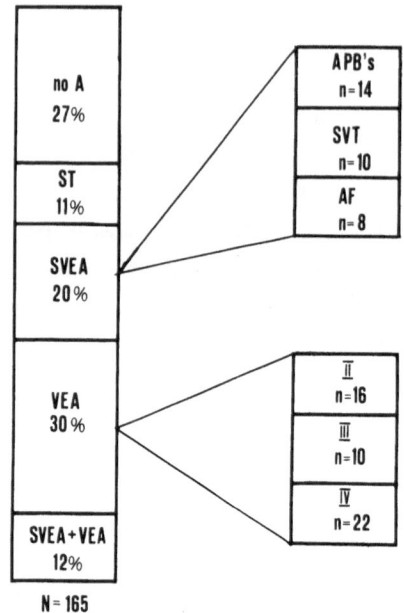

Figure 3. Prevalence of arrhythmias in patients evaluated for palpitations.

A	= arrhythmias	APB	= atrial premature beat
ST	= sinus tachycardia	SVT	= supraventricular tachycardia
SVEA	= supraventricular ectopic activity	AF	= atrial flutter / fibrillation
VEA	= ventricular ectopic activity	II, III, IV	= grading of VPB's according to Lown

Ventricular arrhythmias were classified according to Lown and the highest grade reached during the entire monitoring period was noted. When analyzed in this way, grade IV was observed most frequently followed by grade II, III and V in decreasing order (Fig. 3).

Of the 165 patients 73 (44%) were asymptomatic and 92 (56%) experienced palpitations during monitoring. The overall number of arrhythmias was higher in symptomatic when compared to asymptomatic studies, due to a higher prevalence of ST and SVEA. Ventricular arrhythmias were observed with almost equal frequency in the symptomatic and asymptomatic group (Fig. 4). Arrhythmias in the absence of symptoms were noted in 41 patients (25%).

3.1.3. Correlation of Palpitations with Arrhythmias. A correlation of palpitations and arrhythmias was observed in 43 patients (26% of all 165 studies or 47% of 92 symptomatic studies) (Fig. 2).

These 43 patients experienced palpitations while the following arrhythmias were recorded: ST in 12 patients, combined SVEA + VEA in 10, VEA in 9,

ARRHYTHMIAS IN PATIENTS WITH PALPITATIONS

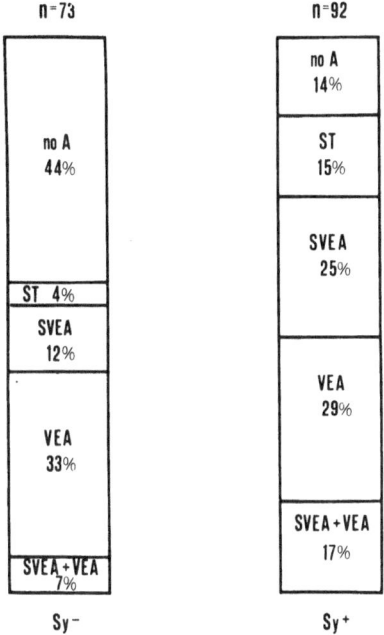

Figure 4. Prevalence of arrhythmias in patients evaluated for palpitations, subdivided according to the presence (Sy+) or absence (Sy−) of symptoms during monitoring. Abbreviations see Fig. 3.

frequent APB's + SVT in 8 and AF in 4 patients.

If one analyzes how frequently a certain arrhythmia leads to palpitations, a similar sequence was found: the percentage of correctly identified arrhythmias was 71% in ST, 50% in combined SVEA + VEA, 38% in SVEA and 18% in VEA.

3.2. Evaluation of Syncope and Dizziness

3.2.1. Characteristics of Patients. 240 patients (130 men, 110 women) were evaluated for syncope or dizziness. The patients' age ranged from 16 to 93 years with a mean of 67 years. The mean duration of recording was 23 hours (range 6–48), and was at least 24 hours in 88% of all studies.

Of the 240 patients investigated for syncope or dizziness 49 (20%) experienced symptoms during monitoring and 94 (39%) had major tachy- or brady-arrhythmias as defined above (Fig. 5).

Twenty-nine patients (12%) experienced symptoms but did not show an arrhythmia. 74 patients (31%) had arrhythmias but no symptoms.

In 14 patients (6%) both symptoms and arrhythmias occurred during the monitoring period but were not related to each other. A correlation of symptoms

34

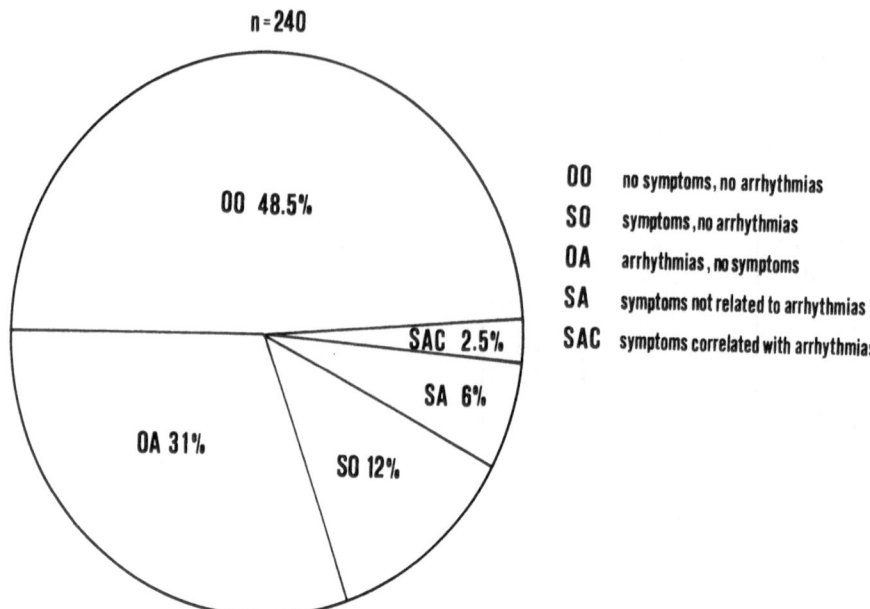

Figure 5. Findings on Holter tracings in 240 patients evaluated for syncope or dizziness. Abbreviations see Fig. 2.

ARRHYTHMIAS IN PATIENTS WITH
SYNCOPE OR DIZZINESS

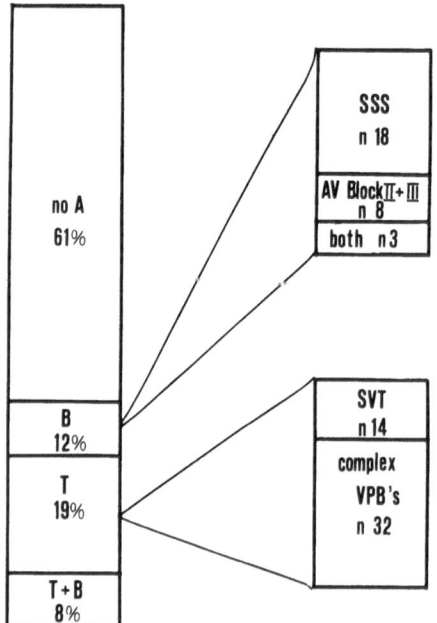

Figure 6. Prevalence of arrhythmias in patients evaluated for syncope or dizziness (N = 240)
T   = major tachyarrhythmias   B   = major bradyarrhythmias
SSS = sick sinus syndrome
Other abbreviations as in Fig. 3.

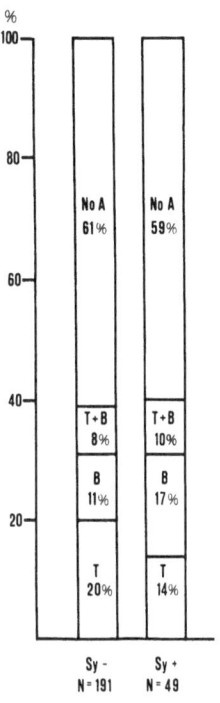

Figure 7. Prevalence of arrhythmias in patients evaluated for syncope or dizziness, subdivided according to the presence (Sy+) or absence (Sy−) of symptoms during monitoring. Abbreviations as in Fig. 6.

and arrhythmias was observed in 6 patients only (2,5%) of all or 12% of symptomatic studies) (Fig. 5).

3.2.2. Arrhythmias in Patients Evaluated for Syncope and Dizziness. In 146 of the 240 patients (61%) no arrhythmias were observed. 46 patients (19%) showed tachy-arrhythmias alone, 29 patients (12%) brady-arrhythmias alone and 19 patients (8%) tachy- and brady-arrhythmias, including 6 patients with atrial fibrillation. Brady-arrhythmias were caused by sinus bradycardia in 5, SA block or sinus arrest in 13, and by second or third degree AV block in 8 patients. An additional 3 patients had combined AV and sinus node disease (Fig. 6).

The majority of tachy-arrhythmias were complex VPB's (Lown grade IV) which were seen in 32 patients, while SVT was seen in 14 patients only (Fig. 6).

The incidence of arrhythmias and the proportion of tachy- or brady-arrhythmias was essentially the same in symptomatic and asymptomatic studies (Fig. 7).

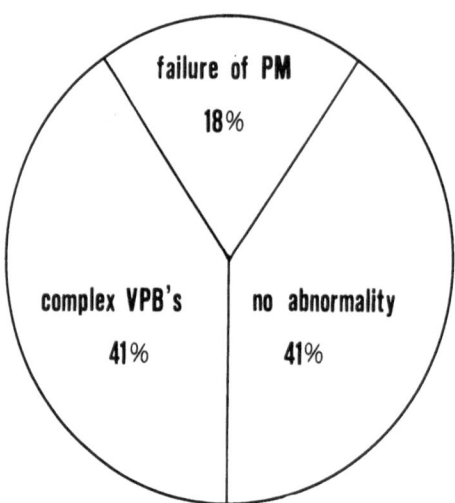

Figure 8. Findings on Holter tracings in 22 patients evaluated for syncope or dizziness despite artificial pacing.

3.3. Syncope or Dizziness Despite Artificial Pacemaker

A subgroup of 22 patients was evaluated by Holter monitoring for persisting syncope or dizziness after a permanent pacemaker was inserted because of a previously documented brady-arrhythmia and/or a history of typical syncope. In this group we found pacemaker failure in 4, complex VPB's in 9 and no abnormality in 9 patients (Fig. 8).

4. Discussion

In our study the duration of ECG monitoring was 24 hours or more in over 80% of patients. In a recent paper, Kennedy et al. (9) reported that 80% of major arrhythmias were detected during the first 24 of a total of 48 monitoring hours. Thus, it can be assumed that the majority of relevant arrhythmias were detected in our population.

4.1. Yield of Holter Monitoring

In our study, symptoms did occur during 56% of the tracings performed for palpitations but only during 20% of those performed for syncope or dizziness. Previously reported figures correspond fairly well with our results and give a percentage of diagnostic studies in the range of 57–94% in palpitations and of 42–49% in syncope or dizziness (Table 1 and 2).

Major arrhythmias correlating with symptoms were observed in 47% of symptomatic studies performed for the evaluation of palpitations which is in agreement with data from the literature (10–61%, Table 1). In patients evaluated for syncope or dizziness, we found fewer symptoms correlated with arrhythmias (12% of symptomatic studies) compared with the studies done in patients with palpitations. Low correlation figures in this situation have also been shown by previous authors (5–22%) (Table 2). This is obviously due to the rarer occurrence of the symptoms evaluated.

The number of false-positive studies (8–12%) found in our patients with palpitations or alterations of consciousness is smaller than in previous reports (11–44%). This might be because our patients filled out their diaries less carefully. The number of false-negative studies (25–31%) lies well within the range reported in the literature (6–50%) (Table 1 and 2) (ref. see Tables 1 and 2).

Table 1. Yield of Holter Monitoring in Palpitations.

Author	Ref	Total N	Arrhythmias without symptoms		Symptoms without arrhythmias		Symptom. studies		Sy. correl. w. arrhyth.	
			N	%	N	%	N	%	N	%*
Zeldis	6	165	35	(21)	59	(36)	94	(57)	35	(37)
Hasin	10	119	7	(6)	24	(20)	112	(94)	73	(61)
Monahan	11						24		6	(25)
Grodman	12	40	6	(15)			26	(65)	11	(42)
Kunz	13	167			19	(11)	167	(100)		(10)
present study	–	165	41	(25)	13	(8)	92	(56)	43	(47)

Table 2. Yield of Holter Monitoring in Syncope or Dizziness.

Author	Ref	Total N	Arrhythmias without symptoms		Symptoms without arrhythmias		Symptom. studies		Sy. correl. w. arrhyth.	
			N	%	N	%	N	%	N	%*
Zeldis	6	158	33	(21)	61	(39)	78	(49)	17	(22)
Clark	7	98	49	(50)	18	(44)	41	(42)	2	(5)
Grodman	12	– –	– –		– –		10		1	(10)
present study	–	240	74	(31)	29	(12)	49	(20)	6	(12)

* Percent of symptomatic studies.

4.2. Prevalence of Arrhythmias

In patients evaluated for palpitations, the leading type of dysrhythmias were VPB's, mostly couplets. It must be emphasized that rare VPB's (less than 30/h) were classified as no arrhythmia in our study. However, less frequently occurring arrhythmias such as ST and combined SVEA + VEA were percepted far better by our patients. The reason for the increased awareness of heart action may be the high adrenergic state often associated with ST.

In patients evaluated for syncope or dizziness we found tachy-arrhythmias either alone or in combination with brady-arrhythmias to be at least as common as brady-arrhythmias alone. A higher prevalence of tachy-arrhythmias as opposed to brady-arrhythmias in this group of patients was also reported by other authors (7). Among tachy-arrhythmias, again complex VPB's were the most frequently recorded abnormality (Fig. 9). Among brady-arrhythmias the leading abnormality was the manifestation of a sick sinus node.

In those patients who continued to have syncope or dizziness after the implantation of a permanent pacemaker for a documented brady-arrhythmia, a high prevalence of VEA (41%) was found on Holter monitoring. Indeed, Bleifer et al. (14) similarly reported an equal number of VEA and PM failure in patients with continuing syncope or dizziness after PM implantation.

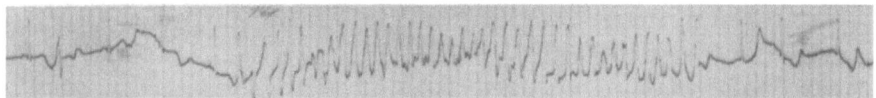

Figure 9. A case of syncope occurring during a bout of ventricular fibrillation lasting 10 sec. in a 82-year old woman who had additional asymptomatic brady-arrhythmias.

5. Conclusions

a. The absence of palpitations in the history of a cardiac patient does not by any means exclude the presence of arrhythmias (6–50% false-negative Holter studies in the literature).

b. The presence of palpitations in the history of a cardiac patient does not necessarily indicate the presence of cardiac arrhythmias (8–44% false-positive Holter studies).

c. Sinus tachycardia, combined SVEA + VEA, SVEA alone and VEA alone in decreasing order of frequency are the most likely perceived arrhythmias.

d. In patients evaluated for syncope or dizziness, tachy-arrhythmias are as frequently found as brady-arrhythmias.

e. The overall yield of Holter monitoring is fairly good in the evaluation of palpitations provided that accurate diaries are kept by the patients (symptoms correlated with arrhythmias in 47% of symptomatic studies). The results are somewhat less rewarding in patients evaluated for syncope or dizziness (symptoms correlated with arrhythmias in 12% of symptomatic studies), but in these patients VT as the reason for syncope or dizziness should always be excluded by Holter monitoring.

f. A substantial proportion (41%) of patients presenting with syncope or dizziness despite pacemaker implantation suffer from high grade ventricular ectopy. These patients should receive antiarrhythmic drug treatment.

References

1. Harrison DC, Fitzgerald JW, Winkle RA: Ambulatory electrocardiography for diagnosis and treatment of cardiac arrhythmias. N Engl J Med 294: 373–380, 1976.
2. Lipski J, Cohen L, Espinoza J et al: Value of Holter monitoring in assessing cardiac arrhythmias in symptomatic patients. AM J Cardiol 37: 102–107, 1976.
3. Bordoulas H, Dalamangas G, Schaal SF et al: Superiority of 24-hour monitoring over multistage exercise testing for evaluation of syncope. Circulation 54 suppl 2: 9, 1976.
4. Hetzeanu H, Yahini JH, Neufeld NH: Holter monitoring in dizziness and syncope. Acta Cardiol 34: 375–383, 1979.
5. Walter PF, Reid SD, Kass Wenger N: Transient cerebral ischemia due to arrhythmia. Ann Int Med 72: 471–474, 1970.
6. Zeldis SM, Levine BJ, Michelson EL et al: Cardiovascular Complaints: Correlation with cardiac arrhythmias on 24-hour electrocardiographic monitoring. Chest 78: 456–462, 1978.
7. Clark PI, Glasser SP, Spots E: Arrhythmias detected by ambulatory monitoring. Lack of correlation with symptoms of dizziness and syncope. Chest 77: 722–725, 1980.
8. Braunwald E (ed.). Heart Disease, p. 796. Philadelphia, WB Saunders Co., 1980.
9. Kennedy HL, Chandra V, Sayther KL et al: Effectiveness of increasing hours of continuous ambulatory electrocardiography in detecting maximal ventricular ectopy. Am J Cardiol 42: 925–930, 1978.
10. Hasin Y, David D, Rogel S: Diagnostic and therapeutic assessment by telephone electrocardiographic monitoring of ambulatory patients. Brit Med J II: 609–612, 1976.
11. Monahan JP et al: Portable Electrocardiographic monitoring. Arch Int Med 135: 1188, 1975.
12. Grodman RS, Capone RJ, Most AS: Arrhythmia surveillance by transtelephonic monitoring: Comparison with Holter monitoring in symptomatic ambulatory patients. Am Heart j 98: 459–464, 1979.
13. Kunz G, Raeder E, Burckhardt D: What does the symptom "palpitation" mean? Correlation between symptoms and the presence of cardiac arrhythmias in the ambulatory ECG. Z Kardiol 66: 138–141, 1977.
14. Bleifer SB, Bleifer DJ, Hansmann DR et al: Diagnosis of occult Arrhythmias by Holter Electrocardiography. Prog Cardiovasc Dis 16: 569–599, 1974.

Mailing address:

Prof. D. Burckhardt
Division of Cardiology
University Hospital
Petersgraben 4
4031 *Basel*/Switzerland

CLINICAL RELEVANCE OF SUPRAVENTRICULAR ARRHYTHMIAS DETECTED BY HOLTER ELECTROCARDIOGRAPHY

J.F. LECLERCQ, R. SLAMA

The development of the Holter's technique often permits to answer to certain questions, but can also create some other problems. Several systematic studies on asymptomatic patients reveal that atrial arrhythmias are frequent. So the disvoery of an atrial arrhythmia on an Holter ECG record is not automatically an abnormality, and the clinical relevance of these atrial arrhythmias should be considered with caution.

1. Detection of Atrial Arrhythmias in Asymptomatic Patients.

1.1. The prevalence of sinus pauses in healthy subjects has been studied by several authors (1 to 4). In all these studies, sinus pauses of duration between 1.5 and 2 secondes appear very frequent, especially in young people (about 2/3 of patients under 30 years), but three important facts should be pointed out: − in aged patients (more than 65 years old), sinus pauses appear more rarely: less than 20% of the patients; − sinus pauses longer than 2 secondes are very unusual (less than 5%) and occur only in young people; − almost all these sinus pauses occur at night, when the physiological vagal tone is highest.

Thus, in asymptomatic patients, it is rarely possible to assess that a sinus pause occurring during the sleep is abnormal. In younger patients, very long pauses may be sometimes encountered if Holter ECG is performed systematically. Figure 1 shows the longest sinus pauses we recorded in a 25 years old patient with a typical chest pain, but without any history of syncope or dizziness. These very long pauses occurred at night (5 a.m.) and were accompagnied by AV block. The association of sinus pauses and AV block at the end of the night clearly suggests an increase in vagal tone.

In daytime, none abnormal sinus rate or AV conduction disturbance could be evidenced. None therapeutic was proposed and the patient remains symptom-free with 2 years of follow-up.

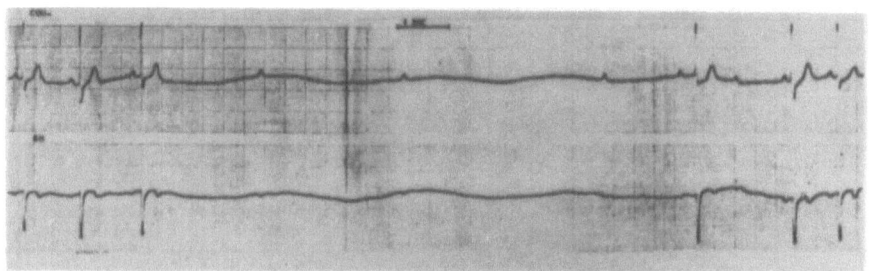

Figure 1. Holter ECG (2 channels) in a young healthy patient without syncope nor dizziness, showing at 5 a.m. The occurrence of sinus pauses coexisting with AV block.

1.2. Systematic studies performed in healthy patients reveal the possibility of premature atrial depolarizations (PADs), with different frequencies as seen in table 1 (3 to 8).

Table 1.

Author	year	age	n	PAD	PAD > 100/day	salvos	PAT
Brodsky	77	23–27	50	56%	2%	–	–
Djiane	79	30	29	17%	–	–	–
		30–57	21	31%	–	5%	36%
		65	25	92%	20%	52%	36%
Verbaan	78	20–80	74	73%	8%	?	12%
Goulding	78	35	20	5%	–	–	
		35–65	60	7%	3%	2%	?
		65	20	35%	25%	–	
Camm	78	75	106	32%	?	?	13%
Southall	81	7–11	92	21%	–	–	–

PAT = paroxysmal atrial tachycardia

The prevalence of the PAD in a "normal" population appears then important, especially in aged patients. The discrepancies between the authors concerning the frequency of PADs in young patients (5% for Goulding, versus 56% for Brodsky) reveal probably a difficulty in the diagnosis of PADs because of the high sinus irregularity in these patients. The main important fact however, is the nearly complete absence of frequent or complex atrial arrhythmias in the young patients. In patients of 65 years or more in contrast, a significant proportion of frequent PADs, and also of salvos or paroxysmal atrial tachycardias is evidenced by all the authors.

Thus, frequent or complex atrial arrhythmias are unusual in asymptomatic randomly selected patients before 65 years. The appearance of such arrhythmias in a symptomatic patient is then important to note and a relation to the symptom is suggested. In aged people in contrast, the discovery of an atrial arrhythmia

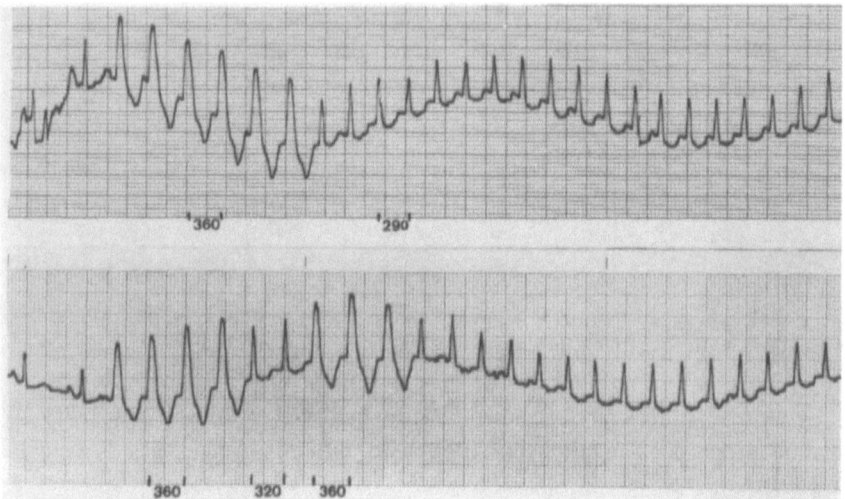

Figure 2. Holter ECG recording showing attacks of reciprocal rhythm. A functional LBBB (lead CM5) increases the cycle length of the tachycardia from 290 or 320 ms to 360 ms, signifying that the circular movement of reentry involves a latent left-sided Kent bundle.

must be considered with caution and have a poor value for the reliability to the symptoms.

The discovery of frequent PADs in a young asymptomatic patient without abnormality of heart examination is relevant, but the significance as well as the prognosis of this fact remains yet unknown. An echographic examination may be performed to search a mitral valve prolapse for example, but angiographic or coronarographic exams are without utility. The description of the intra-atrial reentries (9, 10, 11) with a relatively slow heart frequency during the attacks explain that such patients with this arrhythmia can remain symptom-free for long periods of time.

In old patients, the discovery of paroxysmal or established atrial fibrillation, despite of the absence of any cardiac disease, constitute a pejorative factor for the prognosis, as the cardiac mortality increases in these patients in comparison to controls (12).

2. Detection of Supraventricular Arrhythmias in Symptomatic Patients

2.1. Sinus Brady-arrhythmias

The recording of sinus pauses simultaneously with the symptoms (usually dizziness) is very important. When no symptom is present during the registered sinus brady-arrhythmia, the circumstances of this arrhythmia should be examined carefully: if sinus pause occur in a young patient during the sleep, it is probably not reliable to the symptoms. In contrast, prolonged pauses occurring all the day in an old patient is of considerable value and suggests a reliability to symptoms such as dizziness or syncopae.

2.2. Junctional Tachycardias

These patients usually complain of palpitations. The discovery of a reciprocal paroxysmal rhythm by Holter ECG is rare, but possible. In this case, the relation between the symptom and the arrhythmia is obvious. Moreover, Holter ECG furnishes sometimes important informations on the mechanism of the tachycardia. An example is represented by figure 2, in which several short attacks of supraventricular tachycardia occur during Holter ECG in a patient without abnormality in the routine ECG examination. The shortening of the cycle length of the tachycardia when a functional left bundle branch block disappears signify that the circus movement of reentry involves a left accessory pathway (13, 14): latent W.P.W. syndrome with retrograde but not antegrade conduction on the Kent bundle.

More important practically are the information available on the mode of the spontaneous onset of the tachycardias, which contains often important implications for the therapy. The initiation of reciprocal rhythms by junctional escape beats, classical in patent or latent accessory pathways (15), implies a possible prevention by pacemaker (16). Another possible mechanism is the onset after progressive shortening of sinus cycles, due to block in the antegrade conduction in a patent or latent accessory pathway. Beta-blockers are often useful in this case. Of course, the most frequent mechanism of initiation remains an atrial or ventricular extrasystole, but the Holter ECG is able to precise some characteristics of this phenomenon, as seen in figure 3. In this case with intranodal reciprocal rhythm, as proved later by electrophysiological study, frequent attacks of tachycardia are evidenced in the daytime by Holter ECG. The mode of onset of the attacks is always the same: an atrial extrasystoly is present in the all 24-h recording, but its induces a tachycardia only during daytime (with one exception at midnight), probably because a high adrenergic tone is necessary to obtain a sufficient conduction in the two pathways of the reentrant circuit. The therapeutic consequence is the beneficial effect of the beta-blockers, which combined with digitalis completely suppress the attacks with 6 months of follow-up.

2.3. Atrial Arrhythmias

Atrial arrhythmias are frequently revealed by Holter ECG Several symptoms may be due to this type of arrhythmia, such as chest pain in coronary patients, or aggravation of heart failure.

But the most frequent symptom remain palpitations. The close relationship

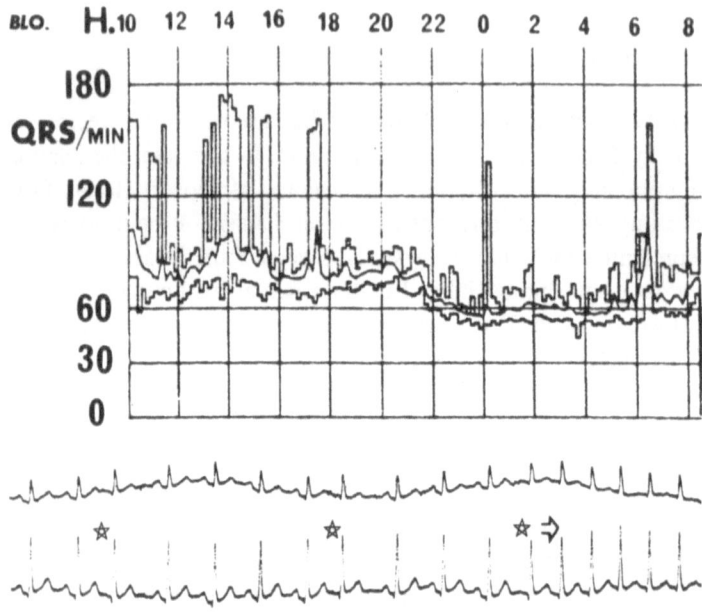

Figure 3. Top: incessant attacks of paroxysmal reciprocating rhythm in the daytime, increasing abruptly the maximal heart rate curve. After p.m., the attacks disappeared nearly completely (only one occurred at midnight) until the awaking. Bottom: onset of an attack triggered by atrial extrasystoly (stars). The last PAD, with longer coupling interval, entails the tachycardia. During the night PADs are present, but not able to trigger the tachycardia.

between these atrial paroxysmal tachycardias and the palpitations is evidenced without difficulty by the Holter technique: usually, these arrhythmias are frequent and this technique is very useful for their diagnosis. In some cases, however, the attacks of tachycardia are not registered during Holter ECG. In the majority of these cases, the recording shows frequent and repetitive PADs. The significance of this fact is then discussed, keeping in mind the high frequency of PADs in the normal aged population. Does any doubt persist, the Holter ECG should be performed until the symptoms occur. Finally, some patients complaining of palpitations exerted only frequent PADs during the symptom.

Moreover, Holter ECG is able in many cases to precise the mechanism of the atrial arrhythmia:
— the pattern of the auricular cycles during the tachycardia is often sufficiently characteristic to permit the diagnosis of intra-atrial reentry. As seen in figure 4, the short and incessant attacks are separated by just one or only few sinus beats.

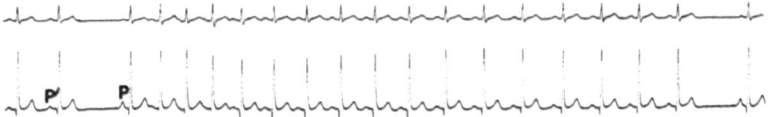

Figure 4. Holter ECG (2 channels) in intra-atrial reentry. The short attacks of atrial arrhythmia, separated only by one sinus beat, showed a progressive decrease of the rate of the tachycardia before to stop.

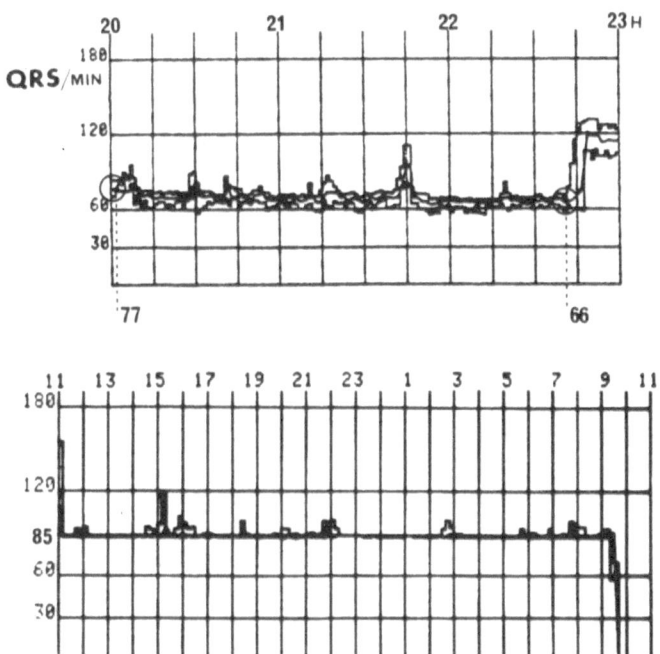

Figure 5. Vagally-induced atrial arrhythmia. Top: onset of the arrhythmia after a progressive decrease of sinus rate at night (from 77 to 66 beats/mn) evidenced by heart rate curves during Holter ECG. Bottom: no arrhythmia occurs after implantation of an atrial pacemaker fixing the atrial rate at 85 b/mn.

The heart rate during the tachycardia decreases progressively before the arrhythmia stops, and in some cases with alternating phenomenon (11). The relatively low frequency of this type of tachycardia (120 to 180/mn) explain the good clinical tolerance. None or quite simple treatments, such as digitalis, can be proposed.
− the mechanism of the vagally-induced atrial arrhythmias (17, 18) is evidenced by Holter ECG. The arrhythmia (paroxysmal atrial fibrillation and flutter) occurs during a period of rest, after a meal, and chiefly during the night. It is often preceeded by a progressive slowing of the sinus rate, proving a progressive increase in the vagal tone. The recognition of this mechanism of arrhythmia implies an

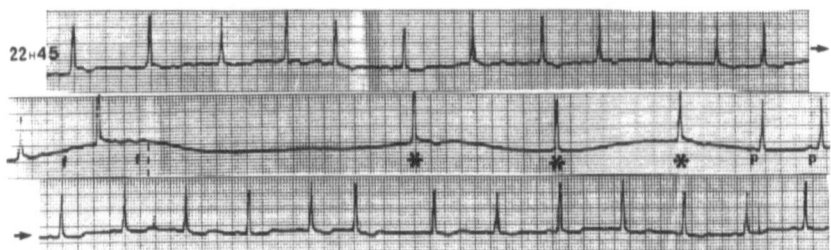

Figure 6. Holter ECG (continuous strip) showing a sinus standstill after the termination of an atrial fibrillation (f). A long sinus pause occurs, terminated by 3 junctional escape beats (stars) before to the sinus reappears.

attempt of treatment with Disopyramide and Amiodarone, isolated or in combination. In some refractory cases with persistance of important symptoms, an atrial demand pacemaker programmed at a fast rate may be used to obtain an improvement in the clinical state (fig. 5), (16).

– in some other cases, at the contrary, the atrial arrhythmia (paroxysmal atrial tachycardia or fibrillation) is preceeded by a sinus tachycardia. Clinically, these patients exerted palpitations in peculiar circumstances such as exercise, emotions, stress, or after ingestion of coffee or alcohol. In some cases an hyperthyroidism could be evidenced. These arrhythmias occur always in the daytime, in preference at awaking. This "adrenergic-induced" atrial arrhythmia (19), less frequent than the precedent one, can be controlled by betablocking drugs.

Another symptom possibly due to atrial arrhythmias are syncope or dizziness. Two mechanism can explain the symptoms:

a) first, a too high ventricular rate, inducing a drop of the cardiac output and a transient cerebrovascular ischemia. In case of underlying cardiac or cerebrovascular disease, symptoms may appear at relatively low centricular rates. Atrial tachyarrhythmias are often discovered as etiology of syncope or dizziness when a Holter ECG is performed for a long time, until the symptom occurs. For Van Durme (20), this represents the majority of the cardiac rhythm disturbances discovered by this technique.

b) second, syncope or dizziness can be due to sinusal pause following strial tachycardia. This etiology, much rarer than the precedent, can be only demonstred by Holter ECG. As seen in the example of figure 6, a sinusal pause follows the spontaneous termination of an atrial fibrillation, with or without junctional escape beats, able to induce syncope or dizziness. But in the absence of atrial arrhythmia, not a single episode of sinoatrial block did occur. This peculiar form of the tachycardia-bradycardia syndrom is important to recognize because its requires only antiarrhythmic drugs, without pacemaker (21). The suppression of the attacks of atrial tachy-arrhythmia entails the disparition of the sinus standstill episodes, and the pacemaker is unnecessary. Of course, the Holter ECG is the need for the diagnosis, to be sure that sinusal pause do not occur in the absence of atrial

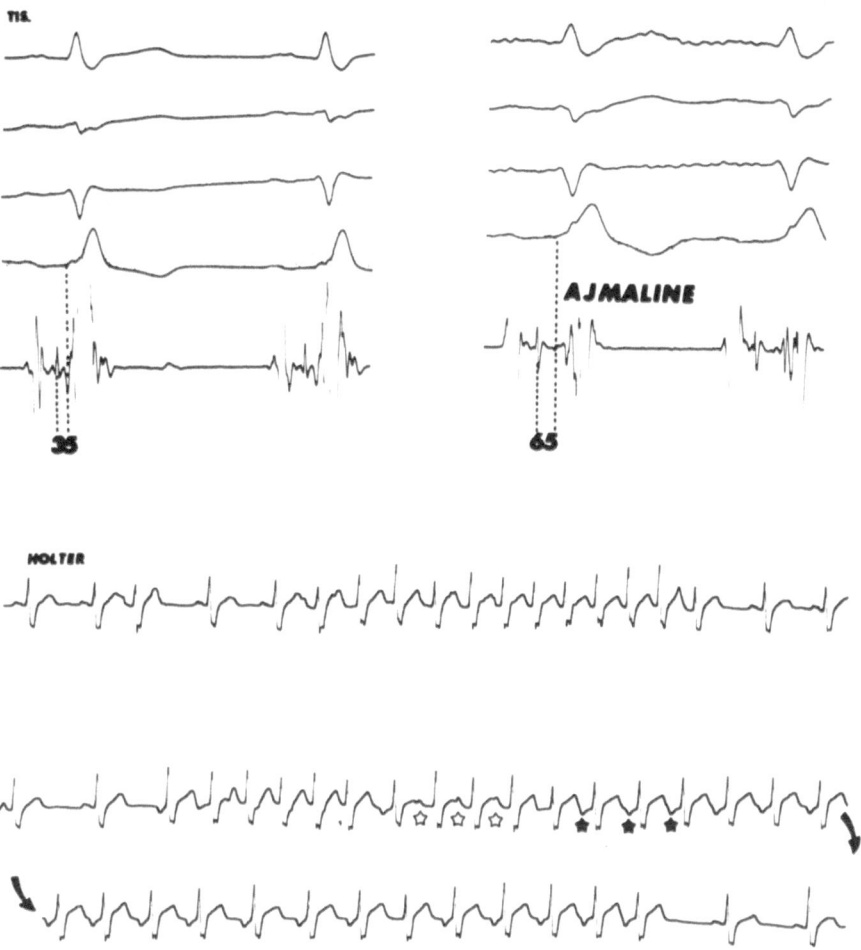

Figure 7. Patient complaining of syncopae, having bifascicular block and normal HR interval: 35 ms at rest (top, left) and 65 ms after 1 mg/kg of Ajmaline (top, right). Holter ECG (bottom) shows frequent runs of atrial tachycardia with two different types of atrial waves (open and closed stars).

arrhythmia.

If the patient has no syncopes nor dizziness during the Holter ECG recording, the discovery of atrial paroxysmal tachycardia does not allow us to be sure that there is a relationship between the symptoms and the atrial arrhythmia. In aged patients with other possible causes of syncope, the diagnosis may be very difficult to precise, as seen in the case of figure 7. This patient, 75 years old, complained of occasional syncopae or dizziness, without palpitations, and had a bifascicular block (RBBB + LAD) on the resting ECG. An electrophysiological study reveals a normal HV interval, and despite of a provocative test performed with Ajmaline

48

(22), no argument could be found for a paroxysmal A-V block. Holter ECG then detects frequent episodes of atrial tachy-arrhythmias with two different patterns, but the patient do not exerted any syncope or dizziness during the recording. This fact suggests an other possible mechanism of syncope: we can also imagine that atrial arrhythmia with faster ventricular rate could be less well tolerated. An antiarrhythmic treatment with amiodarone (without depressive effect on the distal conduction system) was proposed, without pacemaker implantation. A 6 months follow-up shows the disappearance of the symptoms which so far seems to confirm the diagnosis, but of course we are not able to be sure that it is not coincidential.

Another important problem is the research of a cardiac cause in patients after a stroke. Holter ECG is often used in this indication, when none angiographic atherosclerotic cerebrovascular disease could be demonstrated, in patients without cardiac abnormality in the routine examination. Holter ECG is indeed the unique technique leading to the diagnosis of cerebral embolism due to paroxysmal atrial fibrillation, when the patients do not exhibit palpitations. The risk of arterial embolism during atrial fibrillation is particularly high in presence of cardiac disease, such as mitral valve stenosis, but is also possible despite of the absence of any cardiac abnormality (23).

However, a great proportion of patients suffering from ischemic cerebral attacks are aged from 65 years of more, and the discovery of PADs, even frequent or in salvos, remains without value in this regard. Only the appearance of frequent PADs or salvos in a young patient, or of sustained atrial fibrillation in an aged one, constitute arguments in favour of the diagnosis of cerebral embolism due to paroxysmal atrial arrhythmia.

Unfortunately, these findings are very rare, and in almost all cases, Holter ECG remain normal or unconclusive (24, 25). In this indication, this technique appears then as deceiptful.

In conclusion, Holter ECG is of considerable value of the detection of supraventricular arrhythmias, the approach of their mechanisms, their reliability to the symptoms. But the high prevalence of atrial arrhythmias in the normal aged people induces important limits for its use in the research of causes of symptoms not present during the recording, and of cerebral ischemic embolisms.

References

1. Bjerregaard P. 1980. Prevalence and variability of cardiac arrhythmias in healthy subjects. In "Cardiac arrhythmias in the active population" D.A. Chamberlain, H. Kulbertus, L. Mogensen and M. Schlepper edit., A.B. Hassle publ., Mölndal Sweden.
2. Bjerregaard P. 1982. Mean hour heart rate, minimal heart rate and pauses in healthy subjects 40—79 years of age. Europ. Heart J., in press.
3. Djiane P., Egre A., Bory M., Savin B., Mostefa S. et Serradimigni A. 1979. L'enregistrement Holter chez les sujets normaux. Arch. Mal. Coeur 72,655.
4. Brodsky M., Wu D., Denes P., Kanakis C. and Rosenn K.M. 1977. Arrhythmias docu-

mented by 24 hour continuous electrocardiographic monitoring in 50 male medical students without apparent heart disease. Am. J. Cardiol. 39, 390.

5. Coulding L. 1978. 24 hour ambulatory electrocardiography from normal urban and rural population. in "2nd international symposium on ambulatory monitoring", FD Scott, EB Raftery, P. Sleight & L. Goulding edit., Academic Press publ., London, p. 13.

6. Verbaan C.J., Pool J. and Wanrooy J.V. 1978, Incidence of cardiac arrhythmias in a presumed healthy population. In ref. 5, p. 1.

7. Camm A.J., Martin A., Evans K.E., Arnold S. and Spurrell R.A.J. 1978. 24 hour ambulatory monitoring. A survey of active, elderly people. in ref. 5, p. 7.

8. Southall D.P., Johnston F., Shinebourne E.A. and Johnston P.G.B. 1981. 24-hour electrocardiographic study of heart rate and rhythm patterns in population of healthy children. Br. Heart J. 45, 281.

9. Narula O.S. 1974. Sinus node reentry. A mechanism for supraventricular tachycardia. Circulation 50, 1114.

10. Curry P.V.L., Evans T.R. and Krikler D. 1977. Paroxysmal reciprocating sinus tachycardia. Eur. J. Cardiol., 6, 199.

11. Coumel P., Flamman G.D., Attuel P. and Leclercq J.F. 1979 Sustained intra-atrial re-entrant tachycardia. Electrophysiologic study of 20 cases. Clin. Cardiol. 2, 167.

12. Kulbertus H.E., de Leval-Rutten F., Bartsch P. and Petit J.M. 1982. Atrial fibrillation in elderly, ambulatory patients. Eur. Heart J., in press.

13. Slama R., Coumel P. and Bouvrain Y. 1973. Les syndromes de Wolff Parkinson White de type a inapparents ou latents en rythme sinusal. Arch. Mal. Coeur, 66, 639.

14. Coumel P. and Attuel P. 1974. Reciprocating tachycardia in overt and latent pre-excitation. Influence of functional bundle branch block on the rate of the tachycardia. Eur. J. Cardiol., 1, 423.

15. Coumel P., Attuel P., Curry P.V.L. and Krikler D.M. 1976. "Incessant" tachycardias in the Wolff-Parkinson-White syndrome. II: the role of atypical cycle length dependency and nodal– His escape beats in initiating reciprocating tachycardias. Brit. Heart J., 38, 897.

16. Leclercq J.F., Coumel P. and Slama R. 1979. Stimulateurs intracorporels pour tachycardies rebelles. Arch. Mal. Coeur, 72, 1979.

17. Coumel P., Attuel P., Lavallee J.P., Flamman G.D., Leclercq J.F. and Slama R. 1978. Syndrome d'arythmie auriculaire d'origine vagale. Arch. Mal. Coeur, 71, 645.

18. Coumel P., Leclercq J.F., Attuel P., Lavallee J.P. and Flamman G.D. 1979. Autonomic influences in the genesis of tachycardias: atrial flutter and fibrillation of vagal origin, in "Cardiac Arrhythmias. Electrophysiology, diagnosis and management." O.S. Narula edit., Williams & Wilkins publ., Baltimore, p. 243.

19. Coumel P., Attuel P., Leclercq J.F. and Friocourt P. 1981. Arythmies auriculaires d'origine vagale ou catécholergique. Effets comparés du traitement bêta-bloqueur et phénomène d'échappement. Arch. Mal. Coeur, in press.

20. Van Durme J.P. 1975. Tachy-arrhythmias and transient cerebral ischemic attacks. Amer. Heart J. 89, 538.

21. Slama R., Coumel P. and Leclercq J.F. 1978. Les frontières de la maladie rythmique auriculaire, in "Les troubles du rythme cardiaque", livre du groupe de rythmologie de la Société Française de Cardiologie, Corbière Edit., Paris, p. 119.

22. Guerot C., Valere P.E., Laffay N., Lehner J.P., Griman R. and Tricot R. 1981. Valeur prédictive du test à l'Ajmaline dans le diagnostic des blocks auriculo-ventriculaires paroxystiques distaux. Ann. Med. Int. 132, 246.

23. Hinton R.C., Kistler J.P., Fallon J.T., Friedlich A.L. and Fisher C.M. 1977. Influence of etiology of atrial fibrillation on incidence of systematic embolism. Am. J. Cardiol. 40, 509.

24. Fisher M. 1978. Holter monitoring in patients with transient focal cerebral ischemia.

Stroke, 9, 514.

25. Tonet J.L., Frank R., Ducardonnet A., Fillette F., Fontaine G., Komajda M., Thomas D., Bousser M.G. and Grosgogeat Y. 1981. L'enregistrement de Holter dans les accidents ischémiques cérébraux. Nouv. Presse Med. 10, 2491.

HEART RATE TREND ANALYSIS:
PATTERNS AND CLINICAL SIGNIFICANCE

PHILIPPE COUMEL

1. Introduction

The heart rate trend analysis has been introduced in the cardiological semiology by the progressively extensive use of the Holter technique and the computerized processing of the recordings. Not only it allows to detect easily the arrhythmias, but it gives a particularly convenient tool to assess the relationships between the sinus frequency and the rhythm disturbances. The sinus rate is the best physiologic marker we have to trace the variations of the vago-sympathetic balance, and the latter is a determinant of a number of arrhythmias. On the other hand, the presence or the absence of arrhythmias may be related not directly to the autonomic nervous system, but simply to the cardiac rate. Differentiating these two different mechanisms using the same parameter may be difficult, and we shall see some examples of these problems at the atrial and at the ventricular levels.

2. The Sinus Rate

Various parameters can be used to evaluate the long- or short-term variations of the sinus frequency. In the ATREC system (1) we chosed to give an overview of both of them in the same diagram by superimposing three curves (Fig. 1). The entire diagram is divided into 144 periods which represent various effective tracing durations according to the total analyzed tracing: in a 24-hour recording each period represents 10 minutes, while in a 3-hour recording it is 75 seconds, thus permitting a larger or a closer analysis.

The middle curve is the averaged frequency for the considered period, while the upper and lower ones are the maximum and minimum frequencies calculated during the same period from 16 consecutive R-R intervals. A normal 24-hour tracing is presented in the upper part of figure 1, with a general S-shaped pattern of the 3 curves. All the 3 curves are dependent upon the variations of the vago-sympathetic balance in a complex way, as clearly shown by their variations when either the beta-adrenergic or the vagal system are blocked. In the lower part of

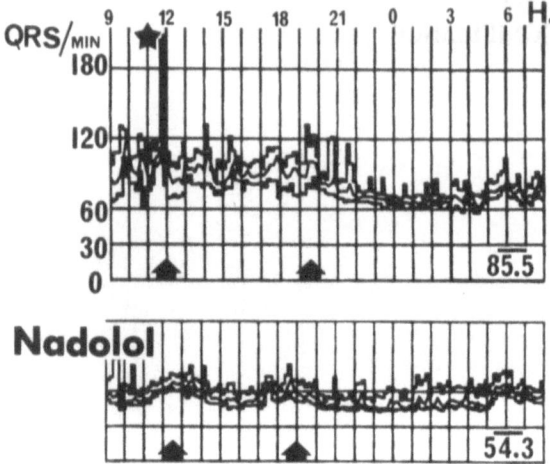

Figure 1. Heart rate trends given by the ATREC system (maximal, minimal and mean frequencies) in the basic conditions and on beta-blocking therapy. In this otherwise normal patient, a short attack of ventricular tachycardia (star) was recorded at noon. See the text for further details.

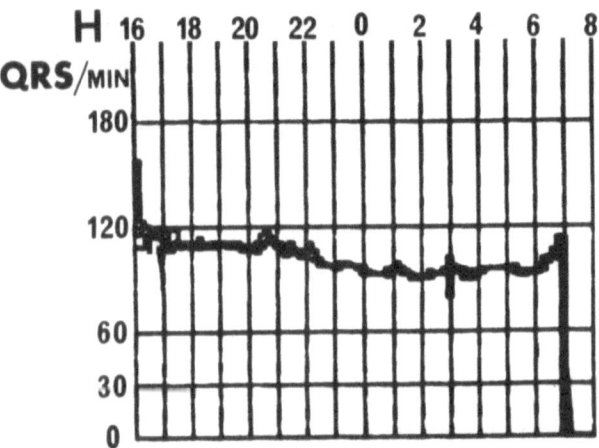

Figure 2. Heart rate trends in a transplanted patient. In this denervated heart, the long-term (day-to-night) variations of the rate are still present, but not the short-term changes of frequency.

figure 1, the beta-blockade by nadolol not only diminishes the 24-hour mean heart rate from 85.5/min to 54.3, but also abolishes its day-to-night physiologic variations. The mean heart rate curve tends to be flat. Still, 2 peaks (arrows) persist at noon and in the late afternoon. In addition, the beta-blockade diminishes the interval between the maximum and minimum frequency curves, thus showing that the short-term variations of the sinus rate do not depend only on the vagus nerve, as classically emphasized. The diagram of figure 2, which is the recording of a transplanted patient, shows that these short-term variations have completely disappeared et depend indeed on the heart innervation, while the day-to-night one persists as it depends on the catecholamine secretion.

3. Atrial Arrhythmias

3.1. Atrial Tachycardia

Figure 3 shows how the runs of atrial tachycardia in this patient are in close relationship with the basic heart rate. Between 4.00 and 4.30am the mean heart rate is at 80/min, and numerous salvoes of atrial tachycardia are present (strip A). After 4.30am they disappear, and the sinus rate slows progressively (55/min in strip B). At 5.30am. it increases again, and when it reaches 80/min the runs of atrial tachycardia reappear.

In this case, as in the following ones, the relationship between the sinus rate and the occurrence of the arrhythmia makes no doubt. But it is necessary to establish whether 1) both phenomena (the sinus acceleration and the presence of the arrhythmia) are dependent upon the same cause (increased sympathetic drive), or 2) the arrhythmia appears when the atrial rate has a definite threshold value. There are two different ways to approach this problem: electrophysiology and therapy, and they were used in this patient. During the electrophysiological study which was carried out also to explore the preexcitation syndrome, atrial pacing above 80/min did not trigger the atrial premature beats. On the other hand, nadolol treatment did control the otherwise intractable arrhythmia even though at exercise the sinus rate was able to exceed 80/min.

3.2. Paroxysmal Atrial Fibrillation

Using the preceding approach in numerous cases of paroxysmal atrial fibrillation, it was possible to show that in most cases the attacks did not occur by chance but were preceded by significant variations of the sinus frequency in various directions.

3.2.1. Catecholamine-dependent Atrial Fibrillation. In figure 4 short and repetitive attacks of atrial fibrillation (stars) occur between 10 am and 1 pm. The first one, which starts at 10.30 am is preceded by a slight, very progressive but definite increase of the mean heart rate from 85 to 90/min. In addition, a further acceleration of the beat-to-beat frequency consistently announces the onset of the attacks (lower strips of fig. 4), the R-R interval immediately preceding the atrial fibrillation being always the shortest one. Actually, this patient was found to have a hyperthyroidism which further confirmed the adrenergic mechanism of the arrhythmia, but this was not the rule in our recently reported experiences (2) involving 10 such patients. In addition to that phenomenon, they had in common their clinical

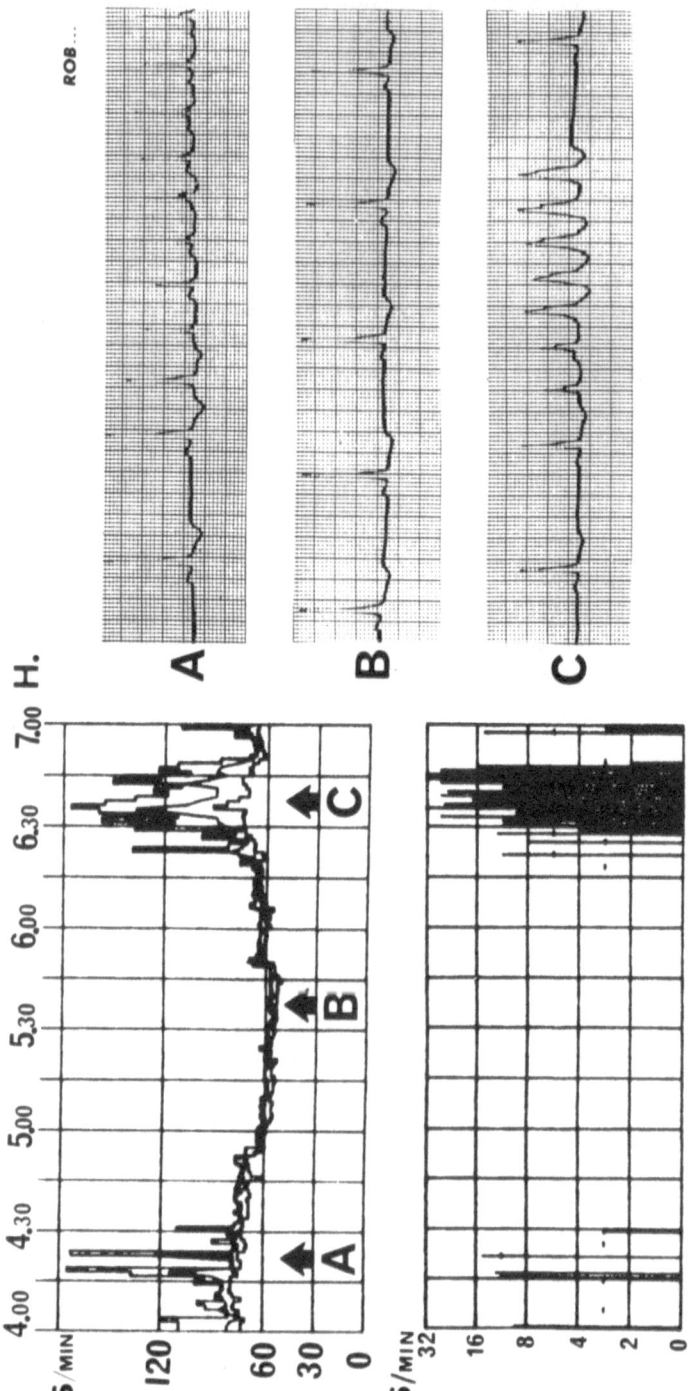

Figure 3. Catecholamine-induced atrial tachycardia. Tracings A, B, C illustrate the corresponding parts of the diagrams: atrial tachycardia with narrow QRSs (A) or with enlarged preexcited QRSs (C) in the context of sinus tachycardia, or slower basic rate without arrhythmia (B). The lower left diagram shows the number of premature beats per minute during the corresponding 75-seconde periods of the 3-hour recording (horizontal tracts for the narrow QRSs, and vertical bars for the enlarged ones).

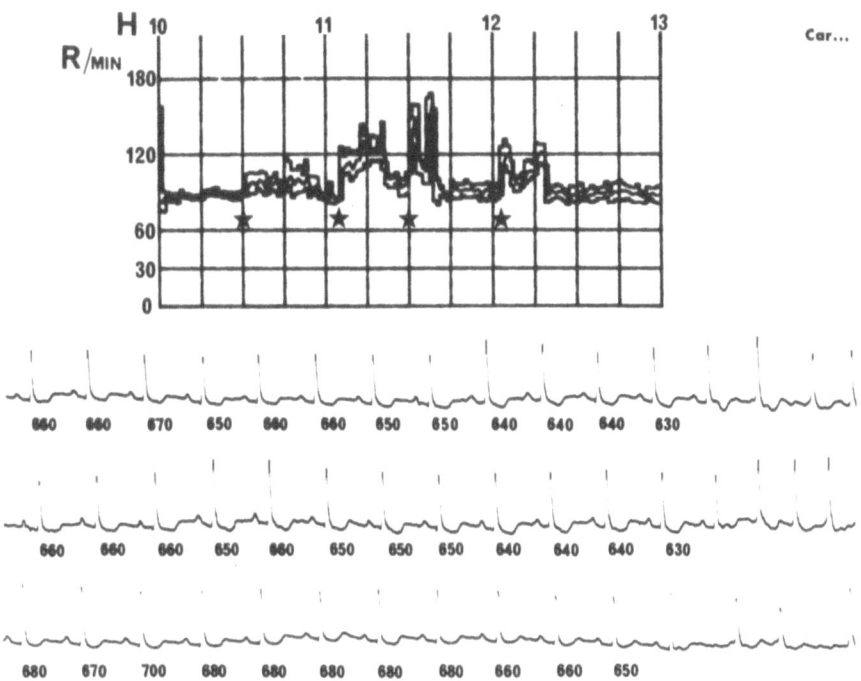

Figure 4. Catecholamine-dependent atrial fibrillation. The stars indicate the onset of the episodes of atrial fibrillation, which occur in the context of a sinus tachycardia (90/min), and are immediately preceded by a further reduction of the beat to beat interval (in ms.).

history of palpitations occurring mainly or exclusively at daytime, particularly in the morning, or at exercise, or during emotional stress. The episodes, which happen in the context of a sinus tachycardia, were variable in duration (some minutes to some hours) disappeared at rest and were sensitive to beta-blocking treatment while they were resistant to the previously given anti-arrhythmic drugs.

3.2.2. Vagal Atrial Fibrillation. The pattern is opposite in the vagally-induced atrial fibrillation, a mechanism which is well-known experimentally (3), and more frequent than the preceding one in our experience (4). Figure 5 shows the progressively decreasing heart rate between 0.30am and 2.30am while the patient is sleeping. The atrial fibrillation starts while the rate is at its minimum. Usually, the onset of the arrhythmia is immediately preceded by a further increase in the R-R interval, with a frequent but transient atrial bigeminy. In most cases, a typical atrial flutter alternates with the aspect of atrial fibrillation. The clinical counterpart of these phenomena is the occurrence of the attacks in the context of a relative sinus bradycardia reflecting the predominance of the vagal drive over the sympathetic one: at night, at rest, or in the digestive periods (particularly after dinner) rather than during daytime or physical activity. The number of the attacks

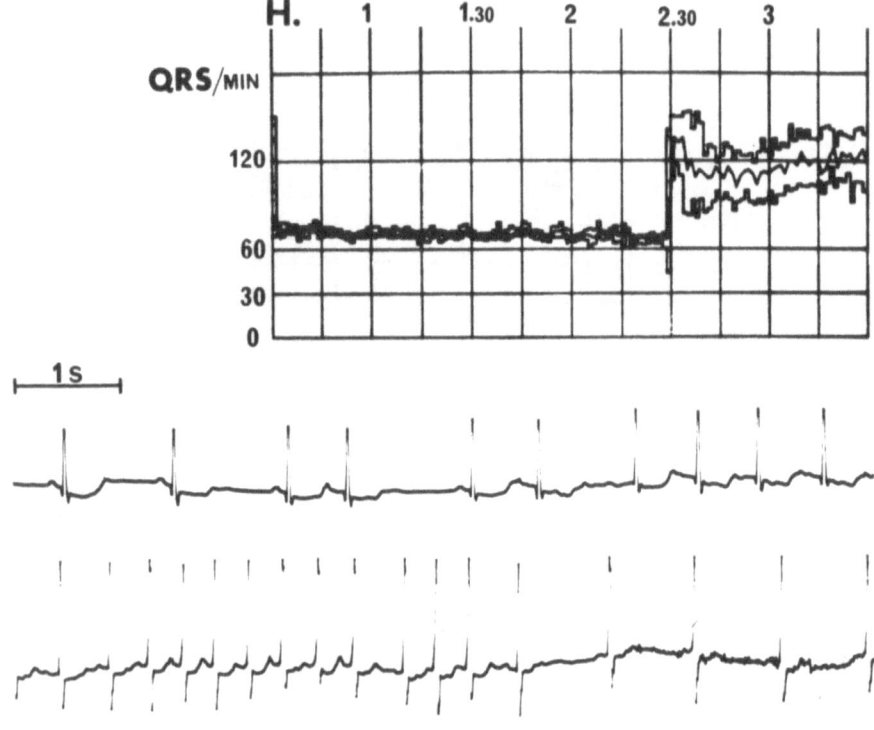

Figure 5. Vagal atrial fibrillation. The attack of atrial fibrillation occurs at night, coinciding with a predominant vagal tone. The mean heart rate is at about 65/min, but the last few beats are at less than 60, the last cycle being the longest one. A typical flutter (with a 2/1 A-V conduction appears after 2 bigeminated atrial premature beats (upper strip), and then an atrial fibrillation which terminates some hours later (lower strip).

is quite variable from patient to patient, from monthly to daily episodes, and there is no tendency for the fibrillation to become permanent. The arrhythmia is usually resistant, and large doses of Amiodarone, given in combination with membrane stabilisers are necessary to control these patients.

4. Ventricular Arrhythmias

The mode of analysis of the trends of frequency is the same at the ventricular level. Still, the difference with the atrial arrhythmias is that the direct vagal innervation of the ventricle remains a matter of controversy, so that apparently the problem is only to separate the arrhythmias which are sensitive to catecholamines from those which are not. In addition, if apparently a very few arrhythmias at the atrial level seem to depend on the rate but not directly on the vago-sympathetic balance,

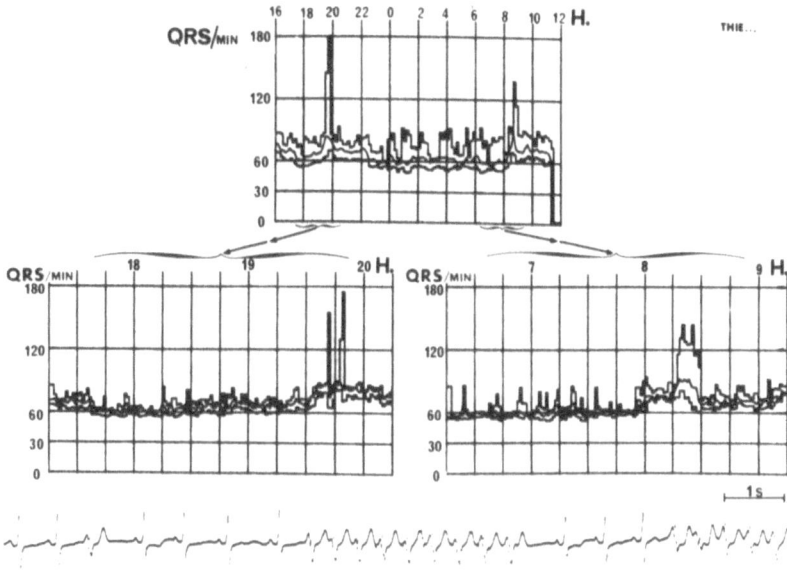

Figure 6. Catecholamine-dependent ventricular tachycardia. The 2 periods during which the ventricular tachycardia occurs are detected on the 24-hour recording (upper diagram) at 19.45h. and 8.15h. But the progressive sinus tachycardia which precedes them is only visible at a larger, 3-hour, scale of analysis.

conversely they are much more frequent in the ventricle.

4.1. Catecholamine-dependent Ventricular Arrhythmias

There is no doubt that ventricular arrhythmias which appear in the context of a pheochromocytoma are induced by an increased level of catecholamines. But this is an extreme, and exceptional example. We observed a short series of idiopathic and severe ventricular tachycardias occurring in children (5) which were essentially characterized by the exclusive occurrence of the attacks in the context of emotional stress or during exercise: here also the link between the adrenergic stimulation and the arrhythmia was immediately suggested by the clinical history, but such cases are rare indeed. Rather frequently, a careful analysis of the circumstances of onset of the arrhythmia suggest the favoring influence of an adrenergic stimulation, but the proof is yielded by the Holter monitoring, on the condition to take into account the heart rate trends.

Figure 6 is an example of the value of the method. In the upper diagram, the Holter recording detects the attacks of ventricular tachycardia (bottom strip)

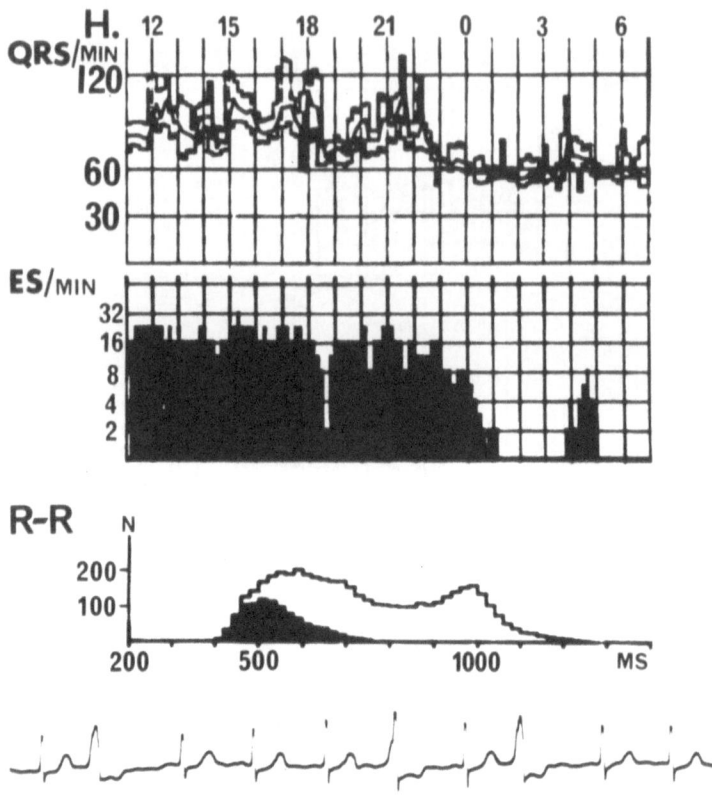

Figure 7. Isolated ventricular premature beats and their relationship with the sinus frequency. Numerous extrasystoles are present from 11 am to midnight, and absent when the patient is sleeping. But they may disappear at daytime when the rate slows (after 18.00h.), or reappear at night when the rate increases (at 4.00h), thus defining the lower sinus rate threshold (see the text for discussion).

occurring around 8 pm and 8 am in this 2 year old and apparently healthy man. The scale of the computerized analysis does not allow any particular conclusion concerning the eventual influence of the sympathetic tone. However, the 2 lower diagrams, in which the heart rate trends are expanded thanks to a 3-hour instead of 24-hour analysis, consistently show that the salvos of tachycardia are preceded during 10 to 20 minutes by an acceleration of the sinus rate from 60 to 80 or 90/min. This strongly suggests the favoring role of an increased sympathetic drive on the onset of the arrhythmia, which was further confirmed by the effect of beta-blocking therapy.

4.2. Rate-dependent Ventricular Arrhythmias

In figure 7 the presence of the ventricular premature beats (at daytime) or their absence (during the night) coincides closely with a mean heart rate of more than

75–80, or less than 65–70/min, respectively. As the arrhythmia consists of isolated premature beats which are followed by a compensatory pause so that the heart rate is not influenced by the dysrhythmia, it appears that the presence of the extrasystoles depends in fact on the sinus frequency, a characteristic which is commonly observed in benign, idiopathic ventricular premature beats. It is very easy to verify the fact during the electrophysiological studies, so that the proper influence of the sympathetic drive can be easily eliminated. In addition, beta-blocking therapy in these cases does not modify the phenomenon.

Still, it is difficult in some cases to differentiate this phenomenon of a lower threshold of the sinus rate above which the extrasystoles are unmasked, from a true catecholamine-dependent arrhythmia. It is why, in fact, it is important in these patients to evidence the presence of an upper threshold of sinus frequency, as shown in figure 8. In effect, exercise, isoprenaline infusion, atrial pacing or simply the normal patient's activity during the Holter recording usually show that the ventricular premature beats disappear at a certain level of sinus rate, ordinarily between 90 and 120/min. The level of this threshold may be apparently a little variable: in figure 8, the threshold was reached at a rate of 120/min, but the progressive deceleration shows in fact that the premature beats reappear only when a frequency of 100/min is attained. This is due to the presence of the compensatory pauses, which make the threshold artificially higher than it really it. Otherwise, it confirms that the ventricular premature beats disappearance was not just an overdrive suppression.

In fact, the things are not that simple. If the threshold phenomenon is indeed a reality, which fits very well with the concept of a ventricular parasystolic focus the rate of which is under the electrotonic influence of the dominant pacemaker (6), a closer electrophysiologic examination shows that the thresholds themselves may slightly vary according to the changes of the vago-sympathetic balance: their value tends to increase for example after exertion, even though the premature beats do disappear during the effort. In addition, when the premature beats are not isolated but in pairs or in salvos, the duration and the number of the latter tend to increase with the sympathetic tone, showing that the repitive activity of the focus is directly under its influence (7).

5. Conclusion

The heart rate trend analysis permitted by the long-term recordings of the Holter technique allows a particularly convenient approach of multiple phenomena which are directly or indirectly related to the vago-sympathetic balance. They are not simple, and qualifying them as either rate-, sympathetically- or vagally-induced is probably too simplistic. But the fact is that they have been neglected too much so far: the artificial initiation of arrhythmias using electrophysiological methods does not explain why the arrhythmias start spontaneously during the patients' activity or rest. By sheding some light on this particular aspect of arrhythmias,

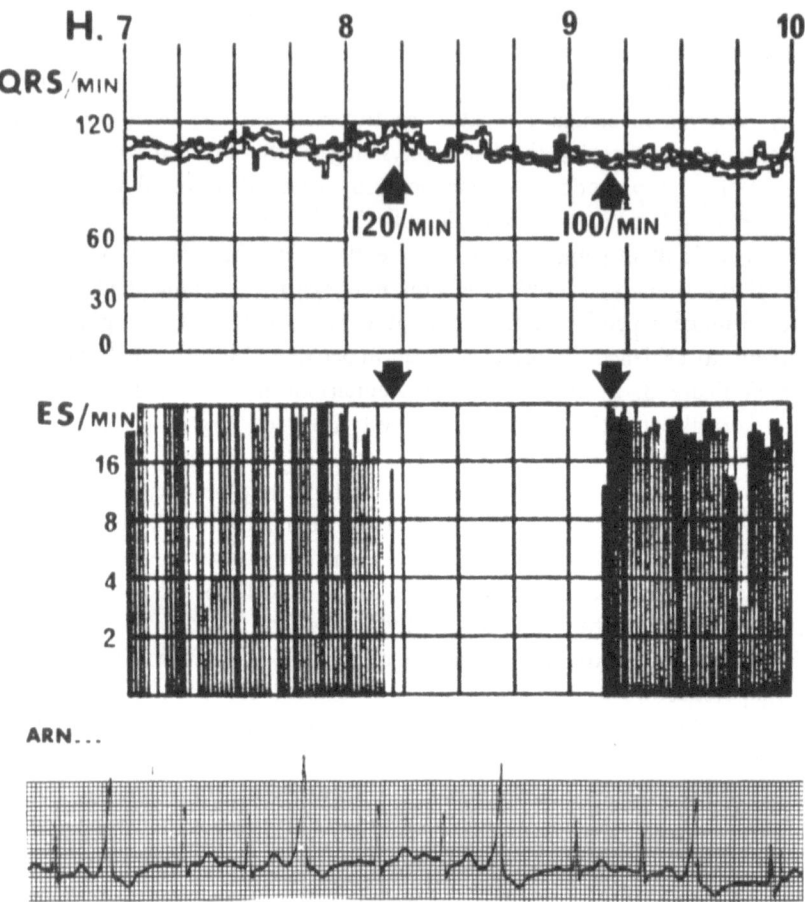

Figure 8. Upper sinus rate threshold of the ventricular premature beats. The extrasystoles suddenly disappear when the sinus rate reaches the critical value of 120/min. They are not masked by an overdrive phenomenon: it should be at about 150/min to do so, as the coupling interval is constant at about 400ms. They reappear when the rate decreases at 100/min, thus defining the upper sinus rate threshold under which the ventricular extrasystoles become apparent again.

the Holter technique is complementary of the electrophysiological one, and in numerous cases it is more relevant in terms of practical therapeutic consequences. This applies not only to atrial and ventricular arrhythmias we have chosed to limit this chapter, but also to the junctional ones: in most cases the reciprocating mechanism of the latter is in fact triggered by the former.

References

1. Attuel P., Rosengarten M.D., Leclercq J.F., Milosevic D., Mujica J. and Coumel Ph. 1981. Computer quantitated evaluation of cardiac arrhythmias. Pace, 4: 23.
2. Coumel Ph., Leclercq J.F. and Attuel P. 1981. Nadolol in arrhythmia. In "International experience with nadolol", F. Gross Edit., The Royal Society of Medicine, London / Academic Press, London, Toronto, Sidney / Grune & Stratton, New-York, San Francisco, publ., p. 103.
3. Ninomiya I. 1966. Direct evidence of nonuniform distribution of vagal effects on dog atria. Circ. Res., 19: 576.
4. Coumel Ph., Leclercq J.F., Attuel P., Lavallee J.P. and Flammang D. 1979. Autonomic influences in the genesis of atrial arrhythmias: atrial flutter and fibrillation of vagal origin. In "Cardiac arrhythmias. Electrophysiology diagnosis and management.", O.S. Narula edit., Williams & Wilkins, Baltimore, London, publ., p. 243.
5. Coumel Ph., Fidelle J., Lucet V., Attuel P. and Bouvrain Y. 1978. Catecholamine-induced severe ventricular arrhythmias with Adams-Stokes syndrome in children. Br.Heart J., 40 (suppl.): 28.
6. Moe G.K., Jalife F., Mueller W.J. and Moe B. 1977. A mathematical model of parasystole and its application to clinical arrhythmias. Circulation, 56: 968.
7. Coumel Ph., Leclercq J.F., Attuel P., Rosengarten M.D., Milosevic D., Slama R. and Bouvrain Y. 1980. Tachycardies ventriculaires en salves. Etude electrophysiologique et therapeutique. Arch.Mal.Coeur, 73: 153.

TECHNIQUES FOR RECORDING AND THE CLINICAL RELEVANCE OF VENTRICULAR ARRHYTHMIAS IN AMBULATORY PATIENTS

ROGER A.,WINKLE, M.D., INEZ RODRIQUEZ

Increased use of ambulatory ECG recordings during the past 15 years has documented a wide range of ventricular arrhythmias which occur in normal apparently healthy subjects as well as those with cardiac disease. In many instances, the clinical relevance of ventricular arrhythmias documented by these recordings and the need for therapy is obvious. However, in many instances the clinical relevance of the recorded arrhythmia is unknown. This is especially true for many of the asymptomatic ventricular arrhythmias. In patients with coronary artery disease, the clinical significance of asymptomatic ventricular arrhythmias is known but the effect of therapy directed at suppression of the arrhythmia is uncertain. In this chapter we will examine the types of recordings available to characterize ventricular arrhythmias in ambulatory patients and examine the clinical significance of documented arrhythmias.

Types of Recording Equipment

Continuous "Holter" Recorders

Battery operated 24—48 hour recorders are currently available in either AM or FM recording modes with either reel to reel tape or cassettes. These devices permit the recording of two or more ECG channels and often have timing tracks to assist in accurate recording and playback. Most have patient activated event markers for correlating ECG findings with patient symptoms and activities. Their small size permits a wide range of patient activities and the most important advantage of these continuous recorders is that all ECG data during the recording session is available for later analysis. These recordings thus permit the diagnosis of asymptomatic as well as symptomatic ventricular arrhythmias. The major disadvantage of these recordings is the relatively limited duration of recording which makes them unsuited for evaluating patient symptoms which occur less frequently than every day or two. They also require expensive playback analysis systems and trained technicians for accurate analysis. Continuous real time printouts in a compressed format minimize the inaccuracy of missing rare events but fails to give quantitative data.

Ambulatory Esophageal Recordings

One major shortcoming of standard ambulatory ECG recordings is that the availability of only two channels may limit P wave identification. This is especially true during ventricular tachycardia when even the availability of a full 12-lead electrocardiogram during the rhythm disturbance may not be helpful in identifying atrial activity. Considerable difficulty often exists on ambulatory ECG recordings when attempting to differentiate ventricular premature beats from supraventricular beats with aberrant conduction. Recent development of an esophageal "pill" electrode system has made it possible to perform 24-hour recordings of atrial activity (1). This pill electrode is 1 cm in length and has the capability for recording a bipolar esophageal electrogram. The small electrode is placed in a gelatin capsule which is swallowed by the patient. The electrode is attached to a thin flexible wire which passes easily through the mouth and can be taped to the patient's cheek. The availability of a filter preamplifier system eliminates much of the respiratory artifact ordinarily associated with esophageal tracings. Use of such a system in conjunction with standard ambulatory surface ECG leads permits accurate simultaneous tracking of atrial as well as ventricular activity. Such a system can be safely left in place for 24-hours or longer without undue discomfort to the patient. The only restriction on activity is that patients are requested to eat a mechanically soft diet to minimize the possibility of chewing through the wires or dislodging the electrode. Diagnostic quality electrocardiograms may be obtained in over two-thirds of patients.

Transtelephonic ECG Monitoring

As originally conceived, transtelephonic ECG transmission devices are carried in the patient's pocket or purse for prolonged periods of time. Whenever symptomatic ventricular or other arrhythmias occur or routine baseline ECG transmissions are to be made the patient removes the device and places dry electrodes in contact with the patient's skin either over the precordium or by holding electrodes under the axillae. The patient dials the telephone number of the base station and holds the telephone mouthpiece near the transmitting device. At the receiving end a decodalizer is activated which makes a short ECG rhythm strip. The receiver may be placed in a coronary care unit where immediate interpretation and feedback to the patient/physician may occur or may be hooked to an automatic telephone answering device and analyzed at a subsequent time. Since patients may not always be near a telephone, such devices may not be able to capture very transient rhythm disturbances. One solution to this limitation is to have the patient carry a small dictaphone and record the transmitter output on tape for later transtelephonic transmission. More recently, transtelephonic devices have been made with digital memory in order that the patient may remove the device from his/her pocket/purse, place it in contact with the skin and make an instantaneous stored recording of the ECG rhythm strip. The subject may then proceed to the telephone in a leisurely fashion and transmit the previously recorded ECG from the device's memory. The major advantage to transtelephonic ECG storage/transmission devices is that they may be kept by the patient for protracted periods of time and thus permit recording of infrequently occurring symptomatic ventricular arrhythmias. They are of little value for arrhythmias which are extremely transient or result in immediate loss of consciousness.

Clinical Value of Ambulatory ECG Monitoring in Symptomatic Patients

Palpitations

Clinicians are often asked to evaluate patients with symptoms of palpitation. This may be perceived as a skipping or fluttering in the chest, a sensation of the heart flip flopping or occasionally a feeling of heart stoppage. Other patients may complain of a rapid heart action which may be described as regular or irregular. Ambulatory ECG monitoring is ideally suited to evaluate the possibility of ventricular or other arrhythmias as the etiology of such complaints. Patients who experience symptoms on a daily or almost daily basis are most suitably monitored with continuous "Holter type" ECG recordings. Patients in whom symptoms do not occur everyday are best monitored using transtelephonic transmission devices. When such palpitations are due to ventricular arrhythmias they may be caused by isolated ventricular premature beats, or brief salvos, or sustained episodes of ventricular tachycardia. Most patients will also have other similar episodes of arrhythmia which are not associated with symptoms. The indications for therapy of detected ventricular arrhythmias will depend upon the exact rhythm disturbance, the underlying cardiac disease and the patient's desire to take drugs to eliminate the symptoms.

Dizziness and/or Syncope

Although palpitations may be distressing to the patient, they often are not caused by immediately life threatening arrhythmias. Symptoms of dizziness, presyncope or syncope as well as grand mal seizures, however, may be caused by more serious and potentially life threatening rhythm disturbances. Many of these symptoms may be precipitated by bradyarrhythmias but transient or sustained ventricular or supraventricular arrhythmias are often the cause. In such patients it is important to realize that asymptomatic arrhythmias including brief salvos of ventricular tachycardia are commonly seen in patients undergoing monitoring. It is therefore important to insist that the symptoms and arrhythmias be temporally related and that recording continue until the patient has a typical symptomatic episode. In many instances this may require many days of continuous ECG monitoring. One cost effective technique is to give such patients old "retired" recorders to keep for long periods. They may be taught to change tapes, batteries and electrodes on a daily basis. Recordings only need to be analyzed when symptoms finally occur. If a patient is monitored until a symptomatic episode occurs and no serious arrhythmias are noted then important negative information has been learned from the monitoring. If arrhythmias are the cause then appropriate therapy may be initiated.

Clinical Relevance of Asymptomatic Ventricular Arrhythmias on Ambulatory ECG Recordings in Specific Cardiac Conditions

Myocardial Disease

Patients with both hypertrophic and congestive cardiomyopathies demonstrate a variety of rhythm disturbances during ambulatory ECG recordings. There has been little systematic study of ventricular arrhythmias in congestive cardiomyopathies. However, several studies have examined these arrhythmias in patients with hypertrophic cardiomyopathies. Ingham et al. (2) noted that 89% of patients had ventricular ectopic beats on ambulatory ECG recordings, 25% had frequent ventricular ectopic beats and 7% had brief salvos of ventricular tachycardia. None of these episodes were symptomatic. Savage and co-workers (3) also reported that 83% of 100 patients had some ventricular arrhythmias and 28% had frequent ventricular ectopic beats. Sixty percent had multiform premature ventricular beats, 30% pairs and 19% brief episodes of ventricular tachycardia. The exact clinical significance of these arrhythmias recorded in patients with hypertrophic cardiomyopathy remains an enigma. No follow-up is given in the study by Ingham et al. In the study by Savage ventricular arrhythmias were no different in the 20 patients reporting a history of syncope than in those without such a history. Furthermore, most of their arrhythmias were not symptomatic and 10 of the 18 patients who reported palpitation during the ECG recording had no arrhythmias at the time of the symptoms. The other 8 patients had only isolated ectopic beats. None of the 19 patients complaining of lightheadedness during the 24-hour recording had serious arrhythmias at the time of symptom. Subsequent follow-up (4) of these patients does indicate that in general these arrhythmias do not identify patients at high risk for sudden death. The lone exception to this may be the patient with ventricular tachycardia, since 4 of 17 patients with VT died suddenly whereas only 2 of 66 without VT died suddenly (p<0.02). The need for therapy of these arrhythmias is unknown.

Mitral Valve Prolapse

Symptomatic patients with mitral valve prolapse frequently have ventricular arrhythmias documented during 24-hour ambulatory ECG recordings. We found that 90% of such subjects had ventricular arrhythmias during a single 24-hour recording and 50% had frequent ectopic beats (5). All subjects with frequent ectopic beats had complex forms such as pairs, bigeminy and brief salvos of ventricular tachycardia. DeMaria et al. (6) also noted a high incidence of ventricular ectopic beats with 58% of subjects having premature ventricular beats, and in most patients these included complex forms. Overall, the clinical relevance of these arrhythmias is uncertain. In many patients there is a poor correlation between symptoms and these ventricular arrhythmias. There is no information concerning the predictive value of these arrhythmias for identifying subjects who will subsequently develop sudden death. The overall low incidence of sudden death in this condition makes it unlikely that these commonly occurring ventricular ectopic beats will be of value in identifying the rare patient who will succumb to a lethal arrhythmia. In some patients with mitral prolapse these arrhythmias do result in significant palpitations and on occasion presyncope. In such instances the ambulatory ECG recording is of extreme value in identifying the correlation between arrhythmias and symptoms as well as guiding the selection of appropriate antiarrhythmic therapy.

Coronary Artery Disease

Symptomatic patients with coronary artery disease are obvious candidates for ambulatory ECG recordings. The major controversy in this disease relates to whether or not routine ambulatory ECG recordings should be performed in order to identify high risk subgroups through detection of frequent, complex asymptomatic ventricular ectopic activity. Although little data exists for most cardiac conditions concerning the prognostic value of asymptomatic ventricular arrhythmias recorded on ambulatory ECG recordings, the situation is quite different for coronary heart disease. There is a wealth of information documenting the prognostic significance of asymptomatic ventricular arrhythmias occurring on ambulatory ECG recordings in those patients with coronary heart disease especially in the first 6 months or so after a myocardial infarction. Most studies (7) agree that frequent and complex ventricular ectopic beats identify patients at increased risk of subsequent death. There is presently some controversy as to whether these arrhythmias identify patients at risk for *sudden* death or merely those at risk for death. Although some studies have suggested that the occurrence of ventricular ectopic beats merely identifies patients with significant amounts of left ventricular dysfunction, available data suggest that the presence of complex and frequent ventricular ectopic beats is an independent risk factor over and above left ventricular dysfunction. The prognostic value of infrequent ventricular ectopic beats, when they include complex forms, remains to be determined.

The major controversy surrounding the clinical relevance of detecting these high risk patients relates to the fact that currently no therapy exists to selectively reduce their risk of sudden cardiac death with antiarrhythmic drugs. However, with increasing evidence that therapy with beta blocking agents (8, 9) and anti-platelet drugs (10) can reduce the occurrence of sudden death, it may be rational to perform such recordings in all post infarction patients and treat those who show frequent complex ventricular ectopic beats. At the present time there are no data to indicate that pharmacologic suppression of these ventricular ectopic beats will prevent sudden cardiac death. Should such data become available in the future, then widespread use of ambulatory ECG monitoring will be necessary to identify the high risk patient and to document the suppression of these arrhythmias by antiarrhythmic drug therapy.

Clinical Value of Ambulatory ECG Monitoring in the Management of Recurrent Sustained Ventricular Tachycardia and/of Fibrillation

As noted above, continuous ambulatory ECG or transtelephonic monitoring may play a prominent role in documenting sustained ventricular tachycardia as the cause of dizziness, presyncope, syncope or seizures. Although early emphasis with regard to the management of these arrhythmias emphasized the suppression of asymptomatic ventricular ectopic beats, at many centers recent emphasis has shifted to the prevention of sustained episodes either occurring spontaneously or artificially induced by premature stimuli in the electrophysiology laboratory. The value of documenting suppression of asymptomatic ventricular ectopic beats using ambulatory ECG recordings in such patients has been questioned. Herling et al. (11) noted an imperfect correlation between asymptomatic ventricular arrhythmias suppressed by an antiarrhythmic drug on ambulatory ECG recording and the prevention of sustained ventricular tachycardia by that drug in the electro-physiology laboratory. Unfortunately, however, this study cannot assess the effect of PVC suppression on clinical spontaneous occurrence of arrhythmias since the endpoint of the study was inducible arrhythmias rather than spontaneous recurrence of arrhythmia. Lown and Graboys (12) have been the major champions of an approach geared toward suppressing asymptomatic ventricular ectopic activity. They report a very low incidence of subsequent sudden death in patients in whom drugs are effective for suppressing advance grades of asymptomatic ventricular ectopic beats detected with ambulatory ECG monitoring, exercise testing and psychological stress testing. Their system of drug administration often involves co-administration of two individually effective antiarrhythmic agents. Thus, the value of ambulatory ECG recordings in control of these potentially life threatening arrhythmias remains controversial. Our experience in use of ambulatory ECG recordings for routine follow-up of patients with recurrent sustained ventricular tachycardia and fibrillation, in whom drugs were selected by electrophysiologic testing, has indicated a rather low yield in detecting or predicting clinically relevant occurrences. However, such observations may not be relevant to situations where drugs are initially chosen by suppression of asymptomatic arrhythmias rather than by electrophysiologic testing.

Clinical Value of Transtelephonic Devices for Monitoring Antiarrhythmic Therapy

We have found transtelephonic ECG monitoring to be valuable for following patients undergoing outpatient antiarrhythmic therapy. These devices are most useful during the early dose ranging period (often shortly hospital discharge). The devices are frequently used to monitor drug safety as well as efficacy. Antiarrhythmic drugs may have a variety of potentially dangerous yet asymptomatic adverse effects which may be detected by routine ECG monitoring. One may monitor the QT interval in patients being started on quinidine or disopyramide in order to detect the occasional patient with idiosyncratic excessive QT prolongation. We have monitored QRS duration in patients receiving encainide and other drugs which cause a marked slowing of conduction velocity. Outpatient monitoring of patients on high dose amiodarone allows early detection of excessive sinus node depression with escape rhythm which may occur in 5–10% of these patients. Drug efficacy may be monitored in patients being treated for sustained supraventricular or ventricular tachycardias. Episodes may occur only infrequently and may terminate before arriving at the hospital. Prompt transmission of the ECG permits the physician to distinguish drug failure from sinus tachycardia or other causes of palpitation. In several instances we have followed patients undergoing therapy for documented recurrent sustained ventricular tachycardia using transtelephonic devices and found that symptomatic episodes were due to paroxysmal atrial fibrillation rather than a recurrence of their VT.

References

1. Arzbaecher R. 1978. A pill electrode for the study of cardiac arrhythmia. Medical Instrumentation 12:277–281.
2. Ingham RE, Rossen RM, Goodman DJ, Harrison DC. 1975. Ambulatory electrocardiographic monitoring in idiopathic hypertrophic subaortic stenosis (abstr). Circulation 51 and 52 (suppl II):II–93.
3. Savage DD, Seides SF, Maron BJ, Myers DJ, Epstein SE. 1979. Prevalence of arrhythmias during 24-hour electrocardiographic monitoring and exercise testing in patients with obstructive and nonobstructive hypertrophic cardiomyopathy. Circulation 59:866.
4. Maron BJ, Savage DD, Wolfson JK, Epstein SE. 1981. Prognostic significance of 24 hour ambulatory electrocardiographic monitoring in patients with hypertrophic cardiomyopathy: A prospective study. The American Journal of Cardiology 48: 252–257.
5. Winkle RA, Lopes MG, Fitzgerald JW, Goodman DJ, Schroeder JS, Harrison DC. 1975. Arrhythmias in patients with mitral valve prolapse. Circulation 52:73.
6. DeMaria AN, Amsterdam EA, Vismara LA, Neumann A, Mason DT. 1976. Arrhythmias

in the mitral valve prolapse syndrome: Prevalence, nature and frequency. Annals of Internal Medicine 84:656.

7. Winkle RA. 1980. "Detection of patients at high risk for sudden death: The role of electrocardiographic monitoring," in Sudden Death. Edited by Kulbertus H and Wellens HJ, Martinus Nijhoff, pg. 275–296.

8. Multicentre International Study. 1975. Improvement in prognosis of myocardial infarction by long-term betaadrenoreceptor blockade using practolol. British Medical Journal 3: 735–740.

9. The Norwegian Multicenter Study Group. 1981. Timolol-induced reduction in mortality and reinfarction in patients surviving acute myocardial infarction. New England Journal of Medicine 304:801–807.

10. The Anturane Reinfarction Trial Research Group. 1980. Sulfinpyrazone in the prevention of sudden death after myocardial infarction. New England Journal of Medicine 302: 250–256.

11. Herling IM, Horowitz LN, Josephson ME. 1980. Ventricular ectopic activity after medical and surgical treatment for recurrent sustained ventricular tachycardia. American Journal of Cardiology 45:633.

12. Lown B, Graboys TB. 1977. Management of patients with malignant ventricular arrhythmias. American Journal of Cardiology 39:910.

COMPARISON BETWEEN REPETITIVE VENTRICULAR EXTRASYSTOLES INDUCED BY PROGRAMMED ELECTRICAL STIMULATION AND THEIR SPONTANEOUS OCCURRENCE ON AMBULATORY ELECTROCARDIOGRAPHY

KLAUS-P. BETHGE, HELMUT KLEIN

1. Introduction

Programmed electrical stimulation of the heart has been used by several authors in order to provoke ventricular dysrhythmias in man. It has been suggested that the occurrence of repetitive ventricular depolarizations following premature extra-stimuli is associated with an increased probability for the recurrence of ventricular tachycardia and correlated with poor prognostic implications. However, differences in study protocol as well as deviating findings support doubts about the clinical significance and prognostic meaning of the "repetitive response" following programmed stimulation of the right ventricle. Thus, comparison of spontaneously occurring dysrhythmias with artificially provoked dysrhythmias as well as follow-up of those patients should provide valid data to contribute to the solution of this problem.

2. Procedure

2.1. Patient Population

The study group consisted of 80 patients of whom 69 were male and 11 female. The age of this cohort ranged from 26 to 77 years with a mean age of 51.1 years. These patients were subjected to electrophysiological study and ambulatory monitoring because of known or suspected cardiac arrhythmias. In 13 of them recurrent ventricular tachycardia and/or ventricular fibrillation were documented prior to this investigation. In addition, 7 patients complained of syncopes. The underlying disease was coronary heart disease in 65 patients documented by coronary angiography. Six patients had cardiomyopathy, four patients had mitral valve prolapse and one patient suffered from rheumatic mitral valve disease. Finally, electrical instability of the heart seemed to be the primary disease in four patients since no evidence of structural heart disease could be detected.

Every medication except digitalis and nitrates was withdrawn 48 hours prior

Long-term ambulatory
electrocardiography   FdB

to the electrophysiological study and ambulatory monitoring.

2.2. Ambulatory Electrocardiography

24-hour ambulatory monitoring of the ECG was performed using a dual channel type recorder (Oxford Medilog 4–24, Abingdon, England) with a frequency response of 0.15–100 Hertz. Analysis of the tapes was performed at high speed (60:1) by an experienced technician with a computer-aided scanning system (Pathfinder II, Reynolds Medical, Hertford, England) completed by means of a CBS-module (Emetron, Unterhaching, Germany) described in detail recently (1). Despite high sensitivity and specificity (both above 90%) of the hybrid computer (2, 3, 4, 5, 6) examples of multiform ventricular extrasystoles (VES), bigeminal rhythm as well as all consecutive forms of VES were validated by visual analysis from ECG-recordings with 25 mm/sec and thereafter tabulated for each patient. Herewith the consecutive forms of ventricular extrasystoles were subdivided into couplets consisting of two VES, salvos showing three to five consecutive ectopics and ventricular tachycardia consisting of at least six consecutive VES.

2.3. Electrophysiological Study

Patients underwent electrophysiological study using two to four bipolar or tripolar electrode catheters introduced into both femoral veins and one brachial vein. Intracavitary tracings from the high right atrium, from the bundle of His, from the right ventricle as well as scalar leads I, II, III, V_1 and V_6 were recorded on an eight-channel recorder (Mingograf Cardirex 6T, Siemens, Germany) at a paper speed of 100 mm/sec with filter settings of 50–200 Hertz for the intracavitary electrograms. The right atrium and the right ventricle were stimulated using a programmable stimulator (Medtronic model 5325, USA) delivering constant current with rectangular impulses of 2.0 msec duration. Programmed stimulation was performed at diastolic threshold as well as twofold, and threefold diastolic thresholds. The following protocol was used in order to provoke repetitive ventricular response (RVR):

A) Single premature ventricular stimulation (S_2) during regular sinus rhythm with progressively shorter coupling intervals until ventricular refractoriness was encountered.

B) Then the first premature extrastimulus was set 20 msec outside the effective refractory period of the right ventricle and a second premature extrastimulus (S_2, S_3) was given with progressively shorter coupling intervals during regular sinus rhythm.

C) Single premature ventricular stimulation (S_2) during right ventricular pacing (basic cycle length 600 or 500 msec) with progressively shorter coupling intervals.

D) Double premature ventricular stimulation (S_2, S_3) during right ventricular pacing (basic cycle length 600 or 500 msec) with a coupling interval of the first premature stimulus 20 msec longer than the effective refractory period of the right ventricle. The second premature ventricular stimulus was delivered at progressively shorter coupling intervals to the point of ventricular refractoriness.

If with one of these conditions RVR could be induced and reproduced, it was accepted as a positive result using the following grading system (7):

RVR-class 0 — no repetitive response
  "   "   1 — 2–4 repetitive responses
  "   "   2 — 5–20 "   "
  "   "   3 — sustained ventricular tachycardia
  "   "   4 — instantaneously provoked ventricular fibrillation ("primary VF")

3. Results

3.1. Provoked Repetitive Ventricular Response

In twenty-five out of 80 patients (31%) no repetitive ventricular response was seen due to programmed electrical stimulation of the right ventricle, whereas fifty-five patients (69%) did show RVR. This was the case during regular sinus rhythm in eleven patients in contrast to forty-four patients during right ventricular pacing. Furthermore, single premature ventricular extrastimuli induced RVR in sixteen patients and two premature ventricular stimuli provoked RVR in thirty-nine patients. According to the above given grading system of RVR the following reproducible results were obtained: Fourteen patients showed RVR-class 1, twenty-two patients RVR-class 2, seventeen RVR-class 3 and two patients responded instantaneously with ventricular fibrillation (RVR-class 4) to programmed premature electrical stimulation of the heart. The latter required electrical cardioversion in order to terminate ventricular fibrillation. In these cases reproducibility of RVR was not examined.

In a total of six out of 80 patients (8%) external DC-shocks had to be applied which restored regular sinus rhythm in all instances. Four patients needed DC cardioversion because their ventricular tachycardia deteriorated into ventricular fibrillation and two patients were those with "primary ventricular fibrillation".

3.2. Spontaneous Ventricular Arrhythmias

All patients underwent 24-hour ambulatory monitoring in a control state. Analysis of the tapes revealed that only four of them (5%) were completely free of ectopic activity. Twenty-five patients (31%) showed a sporadic incidence of 1–24 VES per 24 hours and ten (13%) a low incidence of 25–240 VES per 24 hours. In contrast, high incidence of 241–2400 VES in 24 hours was present in twenty-two patients (28%) and an excessive incidence of more than 2400 VES per 24 hours in nineteen individuals (24%).

According to qualitative criteria of VES ten patients (13%) had VES uniform in shape, nineteen (24%) multiform VES and forty-seven patients (59%) exhibited consecutive forms of spontaneous ventricular dysrythmias. The maximal finding of the latter group was couplets in thirteen patients during 24-hour monitoring periods, salvos in twenty and ventricular tachycardia in fourteen patients, respectively.

3.3. Comparison between Provoked and Spontaneous Arrhythmias

In order to examine the relationship between ectopic activity and inducible repetitive ventricular response we compared the frequency of VES with the results of the electrophysiological study as summarized in table 1.

Table 1. VES-frequency in relation to inducible RVR

RVR	No. of VES per 24 hours					Σ
	0 --- 1	--- 24	--- 240	--- 2400	--- 24000	
NO	1	9	3	9	3	25
YES	3	16	7	13	16	55
Σ	4	25	10	22	19	80

$$X^2 = 3.39 < X^2_{4;0.05} = 9.49$$

The figures in table 1 show a tendency of increased ectopic activity in those with precipitated RVR. However, multifield Chi-square analysis does not confirm significant differences due to this relation ($P > 0.05$).

Further analysis revealed that the group without induced RVR had a mean frequency of 1283 VES (SEM = 548) in 24 hours whereas those with inducible RVR had 3828 VES (SEM = 889) during 24-hour monitoring periods. The difference between both groups is close to the level of significance ($0.10 > P > 0.05$) using Student's two-tailed t-test for unpaired samples.

Comparing results between electrophysiological studies and ECG recordings repititive premature ventricular depolarizations are of main interest. In the group

74

of fifty-five patients, in whom RVR could be induced, thirty-seven patients (67%) showed consecutive VES during ambulatory monitoring whereas eleven patients demonstrated multiform VES, four uniform VES and in three patients no ectopic beats were detected. In the other group of twenty-five patients no RVR could be initiated by electrophysiologic testing. In ten of them consecutive VES were present during ambulatory monitoring, whereas fifteen (60%) did not show these prognostic meaningful arrhythmias; eight of the fifteen had multiform VES, six uniform VES and one patient was free from ectopic activity. Thus, fifty-two out of 80 patients (65%) demonstrated consistent findings with both methods – thirty-seven with and fifteen patients without repetitive VES. This constitutes a significant agreement between inducible and spontaneously occurring consecutive ventricular arrhythmias (P < 0.025) (table 2).

Table 2. Consecutive VES (cVES) in relation to RVR

cVES	RVR not induced	RVR induced	Σ
NO	15	18	33
YES	10	37	47
Σ	25	55	80

$$\hat{X}{}^2 = 5.27 > X^2_{1;0.025} = 5.02$$

Table 3. No. of consecutive VES (cVES) per 24 hours (24h) in relation to RVR

The tabulated figures indicate Mean ± SEM. t = Student's twotailed t-test for unpaired samples. DF = degree of freedom. VT = ventricular tachycardia.

cVES/24 h	RVR not induced	RVR induced	t	DF	P
COUPLETS	35.0 ± 24.1	122.5 ± 45.0	1.27	78	> 0.05
SALVOS	8.7 ± 6.8	23.9 ± 11.3	8.71	78	< 0.001
VT	0.36 ± 0.32	0.76 ± 0.46	5.58	78	< 0.001

In view of 35% inconsistent findings between both techniques the question arise, whether not only the mere presence of spontaneously occurring consecutive VES but also their frequency correlates with artificially initiated, "non- clinical" ventricular tachyarrhythmias. Therefore, the number of consecutive VES during 24-hour ambulatory monitoring was related to the outcome of electrophysiological testing. In table 3 mean frequency of couplets, salvos and ventricular tachycardias are listed of patients without inducible RVR in comparison to those with induced RVR. Due to the marked variance of findings between patients there was no statistically significant difference between both groups (P > 0.05) despite the notable difference in the number of couplets per 24 hours. However, the frequency of salvos per 24 hours as well as those of ventricular tachycardias differed significantly between both groups, indicating a higher incidence of spontaneous salvos and ventricular tachycardias in those with inducible RVR (P < 0.001).

3.4. Clinical Follow-up

During a follow-up period of approximately one year eleven patients (14%) of our study group died, ten of them suffering from coronary heart disease and one from cardiomyopathy. Three patients experienced a non-sudden cardiac death whereas seven victims had sudden cardiac death with a time-interval between new symptoms and lethal outcome of less than one hour. Finally, one patient died after aneurysmectomy. He had neither spontaneous consecutive VES nor RVR following premature extrastimuli before open heart surgery. On the other hand, three patients showed RVR-class 2 during electrophysiological testing and seven patients demonstrated sustained ventricular tachycardia (RVR-class 3) after critically timed premature extrastimuli. This high risk subgroup was further characterized by the appearance of ventricular tachycardia during ambulatory monitoring in three patients, ventricular salvos in another three patients and couplets in one patient. Only three sudden cardiac death victims did not show any consecutive ectopics during 24-hour ECG monitoring at entry into the study.

4. Discussion

A remarkable amount of data have been published about diagnosis, prognostic significance and management of ventricular dysrythmias in man using ambulatory electrocardiography on the one hand (8) and electrophysiological testing on the other (9, 10). However, little information is available about patients in whom both techniques were involved (11) in order to characterize electrical instability of the heart and need of therapy. It is the aim of this study to correlate findings from patients investigated with both methods in order to contribute to the question: What is the clinical significance of artificially induced ventricular arrhythmias in man?

Our results suggest that increased ectopic activity in terms of VES-frequency occur in patients in whom RVR could be induced by critically timed premature extrastimuli. However, several reasons have to be discussed, why our data failed to demonstrate a close relation between spontaneous and inducible markers of electrical instability of the heart. Some are of methodical origin (A), others are based on biological phenomena (B).

(A). Apart from technical details, diagnostic sensitivity of ambulatory electrocardiography in detecting spontaneous arrhythmias mainly depends on the duration of monitoring periods: With longer periods the amount of documented arrhythmias increases (12). A review of the literature shows (8) that a period of 24 hours, which includes complete day and night periods, has become the standard time base.

This gave rise to refer to this period of time. However, one has to realize that with a different time base of ECG monitoring the relation between spontaneous ectopic activity and inducible RVR could change significantly.

Another methodical aspect to be discussed refers to programmed stimulation of the heart. It has been accepted that results from electrophysiological testing vary with time and enthusiasm of the investigator (10). The more so as no standardized stimulation protocol is existing (10). Some authors even change their procedure from patient to patient (13). Our results are based on a strict stimulation protocol listed above (2.3). This protocol was evaluated in a preceeding study, in which double premature extrastimuli at two- or threefold diastolic threshold during right ventricular pacing were the most frequent approach to initiate RVR effectively (14). This is in agreement with findings in the literature (9, 10). However, one has to consider that with a different stimulation protocol the sensitivity of RVR-induction might change and thereby the relation to spontaneously occurring dysrhythmias.

(B) Spontaneous variability of cardiac arrhythmias is probably the most important limitation in assessing the relation between spontaneous ectopic activity and provoked RVR. This phenomenon has been discussed by several authors (15, 16, 17) with reference to the judgement of antiarrhythmic efficacy. Apart from this special problem, the variance of spontaneously occurring dysrythmias has to be considered in the comparison of arrhythmias documented by ambulatory electrocardiography with those initiated by programmed premature extrastimuli. In fact, the spontaneous variability is as typical of cardiac arrhythmias as is the unpredictable moment of sudden cardiac death − and both are related to each other.

Despite of these limitations the tendency of increased ectopic activity in patients with inducible RVR indicates a reasonable correlation between spontaneous incidence of VES and provoked repetitive ventricular response. In other words: Patients demonstrating high incidence of spontaneous VES are expected to have an increased probability for the induction of RVR.

Much more striking is the significant relation between spontaneous consecutive VES and RVR following programmed stimulation of the heart. Two third of our patients showed consistent findings using both techniques, which is in the same range as the results from GREENE et al. (11). From this several conclusions can be drawn:

1. The relation between repetitive forms of ectopics documented in two different ways is better than the more unspecific relation between VES-frequency and RVR.

2. This significant relation has been assessed despite spontaneous variability of complex VES (17) indicating a common denominator of spontaneous and induced repetitive ventricular extrasystoles.

One third of inconsistent findings in our study group might be due to the spontaneous variability of VES. A further explanation of this finding might be the fact that not every induced RVR is followed by the occurrence of ventricular tachycardia or sudden cardiac death. It is of interest in this context that no patient with RVR-class 1 died during a follow-up period of twelve months. Thus, a part of positive RVR-results has to be considered as "false positive results" with regard to their clinical significance. They contribute to the amount of inconsistent findings between both methods.

One third of inconstent findings also stimulated interest in the analysis of the numbers of consecutive VES per 24 hours with regard to inducible RVR. The analysis shows that patients with inducible RVR had significantly more salvos and ventricular tachycardias during ambulatory electrocardiography than those without RVR; unfortunately, spontaneous variability of complex VES prevented a significant separation with couplets. These results suggest that electrical instability of the heart is better characterized by the frequency of complex VES than by their mere presence alone (dichotomy). Quantitative aspects of ventricular dysrhythmias allow a more sensitive separation than their maximal grading (18). Thus, evidence of spontaneous consecutive VES during ambulatory ECG monitoring does not correlate necessarily with effective induction of RVR when they are of low incidence.

The follow-up period of our patients is rather short, but it is noteworthy that with the exception of the patient dying postoperatively all death victims responded with RVR-class 2 and 3 to programmed premature ventricular extrastimuli at entry into the study. Since not a single case of this high risk group demonstrated RVR-class 1 during electrophysiological testing short repetitive responses are assumed to be of minor predictive value with regard to prognosis.

On the other hand consecutive forms of ventricular dysrhythmias were documented in seven death victims whereas three did not show any consecutive VES during 24-hour ECG monitoring (the postoperative death not included). Thus, to a certain extent spontaneous variability of cardiac arrhythmias may prevent identification of patients at high risk for sudden cardiac death.

From this it appears, that a more precise prognostic delineation is possible using critically timed premature ventricular extrastimuli. In view of the unpredictable moment of sudden cardiac death a precise prognostic marker is desirable. But it has to be considered that electrophysiological testing is an invasive method only applicable in the coronary care unit or in a catheter laboratory. Furthermore, with the induction of ventricular fibrillation by this method some patients are subjected to the unpleasant experience of external direct current cardioversion. This was necessary in 8% of our patients, whereas MASON et al. reported about 52% of their selected patients with recurrent ventricular tachycardia and ventricular fibrillation, respectively, in their history as well as in the laboratory (13). Thus, electrophysiologic testing of the heart is a method restricted to centers with invasive cardiological facilities. But there is no doubt, that the utilization of both techniques, programmed ventricular stimulation of the heart as well as 24-hour ambulatory ECG monitoring, allows the most accurate identification of patients at increased risk for sudden cardiac death.

References

1. Tietze U, von Leitner ER, Andresen D, Schröder R. 1979. Ein Langzeit-EKG-Analysesystem zur quantitativen Auswertung von Herzrhythmusstörungen. Biomed. Technik 24, 275.
2. Neilson JMM. 1974. High speed analysis of ventricular arrhythmias from 24 hour recordings. Computers in Cardiol., IEEE Cat.No. 74, CH 0379–7C, 55.
3. Kühn P, Kroiss A, Joskowicz G. 1976. Arrhythmieanalyse – Arrhythmieüberwachung (Vergleichsuntersuchungen von 4 Kleincomputern zur automatischen EKG-Überwachung). Z. Kardiol. 65, 166.
4. Mc Leod A, Kitson D, Mc Comish M, Jewitt D. 1977. Role of ambulatory electrocardiographic monitoring; accuracy of quantitative analysis system. Brit. Heart J. 39, 347.
5. Møller M. 1978. Reliability of quantitative analysis of ambulatory ECG tape recordings. Trans. Europ. Soc. Cardiol. 1, 30.
6. von Leitner ER, Tietze U, Andresen D, Schröder R. 1981. Rechnerkompatibles Langzeit-EKG-Analysegerät zur quantitativen Erfassung einfacher und komplexer Rhythmusstörungen; Systembeschreibung und Untersuchung der Analysegenauigkeit. Z. Kardiol. 70, 22.
7. Klein H, Bethge KP, Werner PC, Lichtlen PR. In preparation. Klinische Bedeutung einer Klassifizierung des repetitiven Antwortphänomens.
8. Winkle RA. 1980. Ambulatory electrocardiography and the diagnosis, evaluation, and treatment of chronic ventricular arrhythmias. Prog. Cardiovasc. Dis. 23, 99.
9. Horowitz LN, Josephson ME, Kastor JA. 1980. Intracardiac electrophysiologic studies as a method for the optimization of drug therapy in chronic ventricular arrhythmia. Prog. Cardiovasc. Dis. 23, 81.
10. Fisher JD. 1981. Role of electrophysiologic testing in the diagnosis and treatment of patients with known and suspected bradycardias and tachycardias. Prog. Cardiovasc. Dis. 24, 25.
11. Greene HL, Reid PR, Schaeffer AH. 1978. The repetitive ventricular response in man: A predictor of sudden death. New Engl. J. Med. 299, 729.
12. Kennedy HL, Chandra V, Sayther KL, Caralis DG. 1978. Effectiveness of increasing hours of continuous ambulatory electrocardiography in detecting maximal ventricular ectopy. Amer. J. Cardiol. 42, 925.
13. Mason JW, Winkle RA. 1978. Electrode-catheter arrhythmia induction in the selection and assessment of antiarrhythmic drug therapy for recurrent ventricular tachycardia. Circulation 58, 971.
14. Werner PC, Klein H, Bethge KP, Lichlen P. 1981. Verschiedene Stimulationsmethoden zur Provokation eines repetitiven Antwortphänomens. Z. Kardiol. 70, 325.
15. Winkle RA. 1978. Antiarrhythmic drug effect mimicked by spontaneous variability of ventricular ectopy. Circulation 57, 1116.
16. Morganroth J, MIchelson EL, Horowitz LN, Josephson ME, Pearlman AS, Dunkman WB. 1978. Limitations of routine long-term electrocardiographic monitoring to assess ventricular ectopic frequency. Circulation 58, 408.
17. Michelson EL, Morganroth J. 1980. Spontaneous variability of complex ventricular arrhythmias detected by long-term electrocardiographic recording. Circulation 61, 690.
18. Bigger JT, Wenger TL, Heissenbuttel RH. 1977. Limitations of the Lown grading system for the study of human ventricular arrhythmias. Amer. Heart J. 93, 727.

THE ROLE OF ELECTROCARDIOGRAPHIC MONITORING, EXERCISE STRESS TESTING AND ELECTROPHYSIOLOGIC STUDIES IN THE MANAGEMENT OF PATIENTS WITH MALIGNANT VENTRICULAR ARRHYTHMIA

THOMAS B. GRABOYS, M.D.

Management of the patient with manifest life-threatening ventricular arrhythmia remains a major challenge facing the clinician. Despite advances in the technology of cardiovascular medicine, we face numerous as yet unanswered questions on how best and to what extent patients with ventricular arrhythmia should be exposed to or undergo various procedures. Further, we are unclear as to how best to utilize these technologic advances in the best interest of the patient with life-threatening arrhythmia. The purpose of this chapter will be to review those methods currently being used in the management of the patient with malignant ventricular arrhythmia.

Malignant ventricular arrhythmia (MVA) refers to a specific subset of patients that have experienced either noninfarction related ventricular fibrillation or hemodynamically compromising ventricular tachycardia (1). Such patients are at extreme risk for subsequent sudden cardiac death (SCD) (2).

1. Ambulatory Electrocardiographic Recordings

There is limited information available on the yield of ventricular ectopic activity among patients with malignant ventricular arrhythmia.

Experience from this laboratory (3) has documented that complex ventricular premature beats (VPBs), corresponding to Lown grade 3–5 (multiform, repetitive, R-on-T VPBs), are both reproducible and a common finding among patients with malignant ventricular arrhythmia. Thus, among 118 such patients who underwent 48 hours of extended ECG monitoring during a drug free control period, 106 (90%) exhibited frequent ventricular couplets and 90 (77%) had salvos of ventricular tachycardia. Day to day reproducibility of these advanced VPB grades was 87 percent.

The surfeit of ventricular arrhythmias among patients resuscitated from out-of-hospital ventricular fibrillation is apparent when one compares the density of arrhythmia between coronary artery disease (CAD) patients who have or have not experienced primary ventricular fibrillation (VF). Thus, while approximately

Long-term ambulatory
electrocardiography   FdB

20% of CAD patients will have at least one salvo of ventricular tachycardia in 24 hours it is extremely rare for this event to occur in more than one hour of the 24 hour monitoring period. This contrasts to the CAD-VF patient who exhibits salvos of ventricular tachycardia during approximately 25% of monitoring hours. Furthermore, frequent VPBs (> 30 per hour, Lown grade 2) and ventricular couplets occur in over 50% of monitored hours.

The relationship of density of ectopic beats to SCD has been examined by Bigger et al (5). While advanced grades of VPBs (specifically repetitive ectopics) were associated with enhanced mortality, the major increment in sudden fatality was among those patients with a high frequency of VPBs in concert with repetitive arrhythmia.

Data forthcoming from Weaver, Cobb, and Hallstrom (4) among 144 CAD patients resuscitated from out-of-hospital ventricular fibrillation demonstrated that two-thirds of patients exhibited complex VPBs, and that the percentage of patients with complex ectopy who experienced a subsequent cardiac arrest was 56% compared to 28% of those without such an event (P < 0.005).

2. Exercise Stress Testing

While appreciated for many years that exercise may induce arrhythmia, this procedure has not been used extensively for either the systematic exposure of arrhythmia or assessment of antiarrhythmic drug efficacy. Our experience in these areas has emphasized the important role of this technology (6–8).

The detection of VPBs during exercise requires some form of on-line recording system, memory capability, or computer storage and retrieval. The use of Trend-scription recordings allows on-line identification of arrhythmias or conduction disturbances. Additionally, it permits the physician to detect significant arrhythmia trends. A comparison between this type of continuous monitoring system and intermittent sampling of events showed a 20 percent increase in VPB exposure with continuous Trendscription (8). Of greater significance is that there was a sixfold increase in the yield of complex or repetitive ectopics with continuous recording. Observation of an oscilloscope screen with recording of periodic rhythm strips does not provide an adequate appreciation of the extent of arrhythmia. This is particularly relevant when exercise provokes brief ventricular salvos of repetitive ectopics which may reflect significant myocardial electrical instability.

Ventricular arrhythmias commonly occur during exercise in populations ostensibly free of heart disease. Extensive experience with exercise testing among asymptomatic Air Force crewmen, YMCA populations, and other apparently healthy groups attests to the wide sprectrum of arrhythmias occurring during or immediately following exercise (9–11). While most normal populations will exhibit infrequent VPBs during exercise, a small subset of healthy persons demonstrates advanced grades of VPBs. Kennedy and Underhill detailed the clinical characteristics of 25 such patients (mean age 49 years) who had had evidence of advanced grades (multiform, repetitive) of VPBs for an average of six years (11). Notably, among 23 persons exercised, 92 percent demonstrated overdrive of their arrhythmia during the final stage of exercise.

The utility of employing exercise as a method for provoking VPBs in patients with coronary artery disease was explored by Jelinek and Lown (6). In all, 1000 stress tests performed by 625 patients were reviewed. Ventricular ectopic activity was observed in 610 of the tests. When the frequency of arrhythmia during and post exercise was compared to control levels, a nearly threefold increase in frequent ventricular ectopics and an eightfold increment in repetitive forms were noted. The most common time for the emergence of VPBs was at peak exercise and within the initial three minutes of recovery. Of these arrhythmias, 78 percent occurred in the postexercise recovery period. Indeed, in the absence of an adequate "cooling down" stage, the immediate postexercise recovery period may be most hazardous for the patient with ischemic heart disease. The authors' experience is similar to that of Bruce (12) in that ventricular fibrillation is more likely to occur in the post exercise period than during exercise.

The yield of VPBs is greater during ambulatory ECG monitoring than with exercise testing. Thus, among 100 patients with CAD, 40% will exhibit repetitive arrhythmia during 24 hour Holter recordings as compared to 20% during exercise testing (13). However, in this same study of the seven patients exhibiting salvos of ventricular tachycardia during exercise, 4 did not demonstrate this grade of arrhythmia on 24 hour Holter monitoring.

There is little information on the results of exercise testing carried out on patients with malignant ventricular arrhythmia. In our previous cited study (3), 76 patients did undergo control − off drug exercise testing and in 39 of 76 (52%) salvos of ventricular tachycardia were documented. Fifty-seven (75%) had ventricular couplets and all patients had some VPB activity.

It has been our experience that exercise will consistently provoke arrhythmia among a small subset of patients with a history of serious arrhythmia not seen during routine Holter recordings. This has obvious implications for antiarrhythmic drug trials.

When we compared the results of extended ECG recordings to exercise testing during specific antiarrhythmic drug evaluations among a group of patients being evaluated for therapy because of malignant arrhythmia, the following results were noted (14). A total of 130 antiarrhythmic phase II drug trials were evaluated. So-called phase II drug testing employs seventy-two hours of maintenance anti-arrhythmic therapy followed by twenty-four hours of ECG recordings and exercise testing. In forty of the onehundred and thirty trials (31%), the therapeutic objectives of abolishing grade 4B, 4 VPB was achieved during drug administration for both monitoring and exercise testing. In thirty-three trials (25%) failure to demonstrate drug efficacy was noted only during ambulatory monitoring and in nineteen trials (15%) *only* during exercise treadmill testing. Hence, it we were to base individual antiarrhythmic efficacy on the outcome of ambulatory monitoring alone, nineteen individual drug trials would have been misclassified.

Thus, the patient may have been discharged on an antiarrhythmic agent that was seemingly effective during a twenty-four hour monitoring session but indeed was not protective for potentially malignant arrhythmia provoked during exertion. This experience mandates the management concept of incorporating both ambulatory ECG monitoring and exercise stress testing in the assessment of drug therapy among patients with known malignant dysrhythmia. This aggressive posture has resulted in gratifying long term survival among a high risk population (3,15).

3. Electrophysiologic Studies

Over a decade ago, the application of programmed electrical stimulation of the heart in order to initiate and terminate tachyarrhythmias was developed independently by Durrer et al (16) and Coumel et al (17). A number of investigators including Wellens (18), Mason and Winkle (19), and Horowitz et al (20) have reported their experience in the use of this technique to define the mechanisms of ventricular arrhythmias and to assess antiarrhythmic drug efficacy. The basis of this method is the insertion of timed ventricular impulses during the cardiac cycle in order to provoke sustained ventricular tachycardia. Antiarrhythmic agents are then administered and testing is repeated in order to determine if such initiated arrhythmia is now suppressed.

An alternative approach — in which the endpoint is not sustained ventricular arrhythmia but rather the induction of single or multiple ectopic beats following the programmed stimulus — is termed the repetitive extrasystole (21), or repetitive response (22). Recent application in patients was carried out by Green and coworkers who studied a series of patients recovering from acute myocardial infarction (23). Among 15 patients in whom repetitive ventricular response was provoked, 11 (73.3 percent) experienced either sudden cardiac death or symptomatic ventricular tachycardia in a 12-month followup period.

Utilization of repetitive ventricular response testing to assess antiarrhythmic drug efficacy was carried out by Schaffer and colleagues (24) as well as the authors' group. In the study by Schaffer et al, 27 patients with refractory ventricular tachycardia were examined to determine whether suppression of repetitive ventricular response by the investigational antiarrhythmic agent, aprindine, predicted long-term drug efficacy. Twenty of 21 patients (95.2 percent) in whom the response could not be elicited following aprindine administration were deemed clinically improved as assessed by ambulatory monitoring and symptoms. Among the six patients in whom the repetitive ventricular response could not be abolished, only one was considered clinically improved.

Horowitz et al (25) reviewed results in 232 patients culled from several centers which employed electrophysiologic testing to assess antiarrhythmic drug efficacy. In these studies, prevention of the induction of ventricular tachycardia constituted an endpoint of therapy. Over a mean followup period ranging from 12–18 months among 128 patients free of inducible arrhythmia, 9 sudden deaths occurred (7.0%).

This compared to 17 such fatalities among 134 patients (16.3%) with persistently inducible ventricular tachycardia.

There remains little information comparing the yield of arrhythmia among patients undergoing extended ambulatory ECG monitoring, exercise testing and electrophysiologic study. Hegger et al (26) have reported on 58 patients referred for management of serious ventricular arrhythmia. Forty-six of the 58 underwent both 44-hour ECG recording and electrophysiologic studies in drug free control state. Ventricular tachycardia was induced in 32 of 46 patients (70%) and identified in 33 (72%) of patients during Holter monitoring. Only sixteen patients underwent exercise testing of whom 7 (44%) had ventricular tachycardia.

The role of electrophysiologic testing in the management of the patient with malignant ventricular arrhythmia remains controversial and still requires intensive study. To date, there is no evidence that this method offers significant advantage to the less invasive and costly techniques of ambulatory monitoring and exercise testing. At present we reserve electrophysiologic testing for the patient who does not exhibit sufficient ambient VPBs against which to drug test.

4. Recommendations for Management

The management of the patient with malignant ventricular arrhythmia requires meticulous attention to the details of defining an antiarrhythmic program which will increase the vulnerable period threshold and preclude ventricular fibrillation. Annulment of VPBs constitutes a clinical endpoint to achieve this goal. While the mainstay of therapy is the antiarrhythmic drug, haphazard administration may not result in enhanced survival. Indeed, Shaffer and Cobb (27) found that 73% of 64 patients with recurrent ventricular fibrillation were receiving anti-arrhythmic therapy at the time of recurrent cardiac arrest. Hence selection of a proper antiarrhythmic program is critical to a successful outcome.

Essentials of this approach have been detailed elsewhere (28,29) and will be dealt with only superficially herein.

The initial stage of management (Table 1) is a control phase during which time all antiarrhythmic drugs are stopped and the patient enters a 48 hour period of ambulatory monitoring during which time a control exercise study is also carried out. This allows for definition of the density, complexity and reproducibility of

Table 1. Management phases in the treatment of malignant ventricular arrhythmia

	ESSENTIAL ELEMENT	THERAPEUTIC OBJECTIVE
Phase 0	Stop all antiarrhythmics	Data acquisition
Phase 1	Acute drug testing	Define effective agent
Phase 2	Short term maintenance	Determine drug tolerance
Phase 3	Long term maintenance	Prevention of recurrence

84

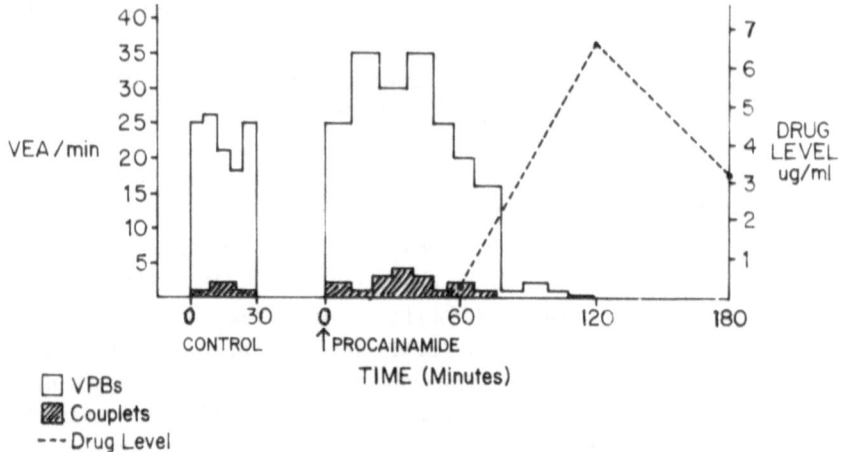

Figure 1. Acute drug testing: Procainamide. After 60 minutes, near complete abolition of repetitive forms (dark areas) and single VPBs. This effect correlated with therapeutic drug level.

VPBs for each patient.

Acute (Phase 1) and short term (Phase 2) drug testing is next undertaken providing the patient exhibits sufficient ambient ventricular ectopic activity and reproducible repetitive VPBs. Not only are several drugs profiled for efficacy but are also assessed for potential idiosyncratic aggravation of arrhythmia.

The acute drug testing protocol involves four elements. *First* is the administration of a single large oral dose of a selected antiarrhythmic drug. *Second* is the use of programmed monitoring (Trendscription) to display the time course of drug action (Figure 1) over an observation period of 3–5 hours. *Third* is the sampling of bloods for drug concentration during the testing. This is particularly helpful if the drug level is low for it then allows for a higher dosage. Finally are brief periods of bicycle exercise hourly during the test to assess the response of the agent on exercise-induced arrhythmia.

Once an appropriate drug is found, a phase II is begun during which 48–72 hours of drug administration is followed by Holter monitoring and treadmill exercise testing.

5. Objectives of Therapy

Complete elimination of ectopic activity is at times impossible to accomplish. It has been the author's view that suppression of repetitive and early cycle (R-on-T) VPBs and elimination of ventricular tachycardia are essential if the patient is to be protected against malignant ventricular arrhythmias.

The following treatment objectives are suggested:

1. Elimination of all early cycle VPBs (grade 5), ventricular tachycardia (grade

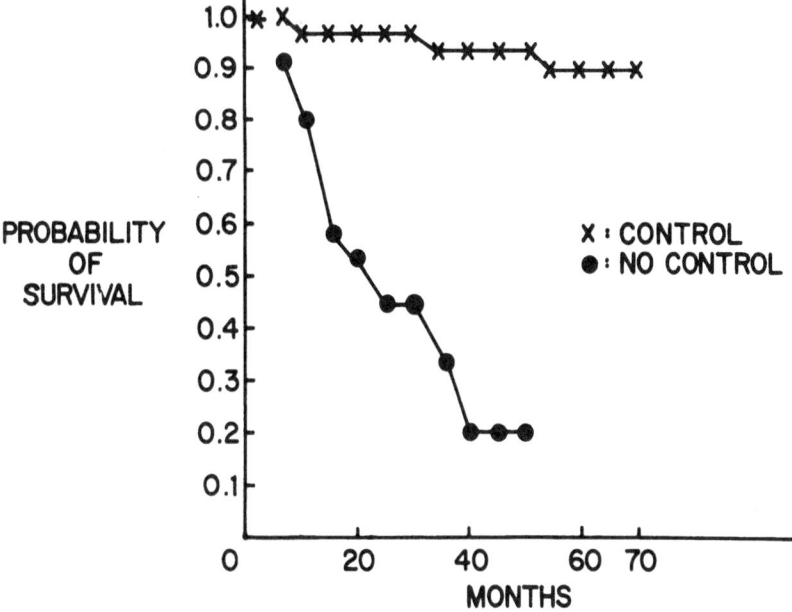

Figure 2. Sudden cardiac death among 141 patients with malignant ventricular arrhythmia hased on control (x) of salvos of ventricular tachycardia and early cycle VPBs or no control (•).

4B), and reduction of ventricular couplets (grade 4A) activity to no more than their occasional occurrence during a 24-hour ambulatory monitoring session.

2. Elimination of ventricular salvos and early cycle VPBs at peak exercise and within the first three minutes of recovery from maximal treadmill exercise testing.

3. In patients undergoing electrophysiologic testing, it is necessary that the selected drug program suppress the multiple ventricular response which had been elicited during control testing.

It needs to be emphasized that electrophysiologic testing is as yet an investigational method. The practicing physician can address the problem of sudden cardiac death adequately by focusing on advanced grades of VPBs exposed during 24-hour monitoring and exercise testing.

6. Does Reduction of VPBs Protect Against Sudden Cardiac Death?

If the presence of advanced grades of VPBs are indicators of the presence of electrical instability, their suppression should afford protection against sudden cardiac death. This then is an acid test of the VPB hypothesis. We have analyzed survival among 141 patients (114 males, 27 females, average age 53 years) with malignant ventricular arrhythmia dependent upon the abolition by antiarrhythmic drugs of salvos of ventricular tachycardia and R-on-T VPBs (Lown grades 4B and 5) (Figure 2).

Over an average follow-up of 24.5 months there were 35 deaths (12.4% annual mortality) of whom 23 patients succumbed suddenly (8.2% annual mortality). Among 116 patients in whom antiarrhythmic drugs abolished grades 4B and 5 VPBs, only 6 sudden deaths occurred for a 2.3% annual mortality. Even among patients with left ventricular dysfunction (LVD), control of VPBs was a critical element predicting survival. Annual sudden death for the noncontrolled group with LVD was 41% contrasting with only 2.4% for the LVD subgroup in whom advanced VPB grades were abolished.

This experience indicates that antiarrhythmic drugs can protect against the recurrence of life-threatening arrhythmias and that abolition of certain advanced grades of VPBs provide an effective therapeutic objective. It is clear that each patient must be managed individually. No single method, whether it be Holter monitoring, exercise testing or electrophysiologic testing will suffice or can be used exclusively. As we do not rely on one diagnostic approach to manage coronary artery disease, valvular disease or cardiomyopathy, we can not rely on one approach to manage the patient with life-threatening dysrhythmia.

References

1. Lown B, Graboys TB. 1977. Management of the patient with malignant ventricular arrhythmias. Am J Cardiol. 39, 910–19.
2. Cobb LA, Baum RS, Alvarez H, Schafter WA. 1975. Resuscitation from out-of-hospital ventricular fibrillation: 4-year follow-up Circulation. 51 & 52, III, 223.
3. Graboys TB, Lown B, Podrid PJ, DeSilva RA. 1982, in press. Long term survival of patients with malignant ventricular arrhythmia treated with antiarrhythmic drugs. Am J Cardiol.
4. Weaver WD, Cobb LA, Hallstrom AP. 1982, in press. Ambulatory arrhythmias in resuscitated victims of cardiac arrest. Circulation.
5. Bigger JT, Weld FM. 1981. Analysis of prognostic significance of ventricular arrhythmias after myocardial infarction. Shortcomings of Lown grading system. Br Heart J. 45, 717–24.
6. Jelinek NV, Lown B. 1974. Exercise stress testing for exposure of cardiac arrhythmia. Progr Cardiovasc Dis. 26, 497.
7. Graboys TB, DeSilva RD, Lown B. 1978. Exercise stress testing and ambulatory monitoring in patiens with malignant ventricular arrhythmia. Am J Cardiol. 41,400.
8. Antman E, Graboys TB, Lown B. 1979. Comparison of continuous to intermittent electrocardiographic monitoring during exercise testing for exposure of cardiac arrhythmias. JAMA. 241, 2802–2805.
9. Lamb CE, Hiss RG. 1962. Influence of exercise on premature contractions. AM J Cardiol. 10, 209.
10. Froelicher VF, Thompson AJ, Longo Mr. 1976. Value of exercise testing for screening asymptomatic men for latent coronary artery disease. Progr Cardiovasc Dis. 18, 265.
11. Kennedy LH, Underhill SJ. 1976. Frequent or complex ventricular ectopic in apparently healthy subjects. Am J Cardiol. 38, 141.
12. Irving JB, Bruce RA. 1977. Exertional hypotension and postexertional ventricular fibrillation in stress testing. Am J Cardiol. 39, 849.
13. Ryan M, Lown B, Horn H. 1975. Comparison of ventricular activity during 24-hour monitoring and exercise testing in patients with coronary heart disease. N Engl J Med. 292, 224–9.

14. Graboys TB. 1981. Limitations of ambulatory electrocardiographic recordings to assess antiarrhythmic drug efficacy. In: Ambulatory Electrocardiographic Recording. Year Book Medical Publications. Edited by Wenger et al. Chicago.

15. Grayboys TB, Lown B, Podrid PJ, DeSilva RA. 1979. Survival of patients with malignant ventricular arrhythmias treated with antiarrhythmic agents. Circulation. 60:4, 285.

16. Durrer D, School L, Schuinerbrug RM, et al. 1967. The role of premature termination of supraventricular tachycardia in the Wolff-Parkinson-White syndrome. Circulation. 36, 655.

17. Coumell Ph, Cabrol C, Fabioto A, et al. 1967. Tachycardia permanente par rhythme reciproque. Arch Mal Coeur. 60, 1830.

18. Wellens HJJJ, Durer DR, Lie KI. 1976. Observations on mechanisms of ventricular tachycardia in man. Circulation. 54, 237.

19. Mason JW, Winkle RA. 1978. Electrode catheter arrhythmia induction in the selection and assessment of antiarrhythmic drug therapy for recurrent ventricular tachycardia. Circulation. 58, 971–85.

20. Horowitz LN, Josephson ME, Farshidi A, et al. 1978. Recurrent sustained ventricular tachycardia. 3. Role of the electrophysiologic study in selection of antiarrhythmic regiments. Circulation. 58, 986K–97.

21. Matta RJ, Verrier RL, Lown B. 1976. The repetitive extrasystole as an index of vulnerability of ventricular fibrillation. AM J Physiol. 230, 1461

22. Barr I, Klein MD, Lown B. 1970. Repetitive ventricular response (RVR) in the digitalized heart of various mammalian species. Proc Soc Exp Biol Med. 134, 841.

23. Green HL, Reid PR, Schaeffer AH. 1978. The repetitive ventricular response in man: A predictor of sudden death. N Engl J Med. 299, 702–34.

24. Schaeffer AH, Green HL, Reid PR. 1978. Suppression of the repetitive ventricular response: An index of long-term antiarrhythmic effectiveness of Aprindine for ventricular tachycardia in man. Circulation. 42, 1007–12.

25. Horowitz LN, Josephson ME, Kastor JA. 1980. Intracardiac electrophysiologic studies as a method for the optimazation of drug therapy in chronic ventricular arrhythmia. Prog Cardiovasc Dis. 23, 81–98.

26. Hegger JV, Prystowsky EN, Jackman W, et al. 1981, Ed. Wenger et al., Comparison between results obtained from electrophysiologic testing, exercise testing and ambulatory ECG recording. In: Ambulatory Electrocardiographic Recording. Year Book Medical Publishers. p. 379–389.

27. Schaffer WA, Cobb LA. 1975. Recurrent ventricular fibrillation and modes of deatch in survivors of out-of-hospital ventricular fibrillation. N Engl J Med. 293, 260–2.

28. Lown B, Graboys TB. 1980: March, Vol. 3. Ed. McIntosh HD. Ventricular premature beats and sudden cardiac death. Baylor Cardiology Series.

29. Lown B, Podrid PJ, DeSilva RA, Graboys TB. 1980, March. Vol IV. Sudden Cardiac Death: Management of the patient at risk. Year Book Medical Publications.

CONTINUOUS ST-SEGMENT MONITORING: INDICATIONS AND LIMITATIONS

MAARTEN L. SIMOONS, MD.

In patients with chest discomfort, episodes of myocardial ischemia can be documented by changes in the electrocardiogram (ECG). Spontaneous episodes can be recorded by a standard ECG equipment during hospitalisation in patients with unstable angina. Exercise testing is frequently used to induce symptoms and ECG changes in patients with stable angina.

Finally, ambulatory electrocardiography may be used for detection of ECG changes during normal activities outside the hospital. In this study the relative values of exercise testing and ambulatory ECG recording for the detection of ST segment changes are compared.

Technical Considerations

Ambulatory electrocardiography is currently mostly employed for the detection of rhythm and conduction disturbances, as discussed elsewhere in this symposium. For this purpose the frequency response of the recorder and play back unit is not critical. Many systems purposely use a relatively high cut off of the lower frequencies in order to reduce baseline drift. However, a correct frequency response is mandatory for proper analysis of changes of the QRS and ST waveforms. A recent study (1) has demonstrated that most systems for ambulatory electrocardiography are not suitable for ST-segment analysis. However, the FM-recording system used in our studies has an adequate frequency response, although, the recorded ECG signal has a high noise level (1, 2). This has been partially improved in newer model recorders (figure 1).

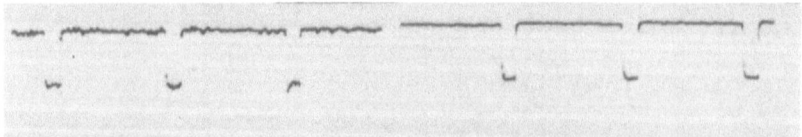

Figure 1. Calibration signal (1 mV) Medilog II recorder. The signal was recorded on tape, played back and reproduced on the stripchart recorder of the Medilog II system. Note high noise level in the recording in 1980 (left) which has been improved in the 1981 version of the system (right).

Patient Selection

For the present study two groups of patients were selected. The first group consisted of 40 males and 5 females who had been referred for stress testing because of chest discomfort. Seventeen patients had a previous myocardial infarction, five of these as well as four others had coronary bypass surgery prior to the study. The second group included 31 male participants in our rehabilitation program. Twenty two patients were rehabilitated after a myocardial infarction and 9 after coronary bypass surgery. The ages were between 33 and 68 years. Medication used by the patients was not changed for the present study (table 1).

Table 1. Medication used at the time of the study. Many patients were on combination of drugs.

Medication	I (45)	II (31)
None	13	7
Beta blocker	23	8
Digoxine	9	3
Diuretics	8	4
Anti-arrhythmics	3	2
Others	2	8

Study Protocol

The patients with possible angina, group I, were asked to participate in the study prior to the exercise test. The Frank corrected orthogonal lead ECG during exercise was analysed online with a special computer system (3). Simultaneously two ECG precordial leads were recorded with the Oxford Instruments Medilog II system. The first lead was obtained between midsternum and V_3, the second lead between the top of the sternum and V_5 (lead CM_5). Attention was paid to careful skin preparation and fixation of the electrodes and cables. The patients then performed a symptom limited exercise test on a bicycle ergometer, with stepwise workload increments of 10 Watts per minute. In none of the patients the test was terminated for ECG changes. After the exercise test the Frank leads were disconnected. Ambulatory ECG recording continued for 24 hours of normal activities outside the hospital.

The participants in the rehabilitation program, group II, underwent ambulatory monitoring with the same equipment and leads during two consecutive days. That period included one rehabilitation session of approximately 90 minutes. At the end of the 48 hour recording period each patient performed an exercise test, similar to group I. The electrodes and cables were checked before the exercise test. All patients kept a diary of activities and symptoms during monitoring.

The ambulatory ECG recordings were analysed at 60 x normal speed with

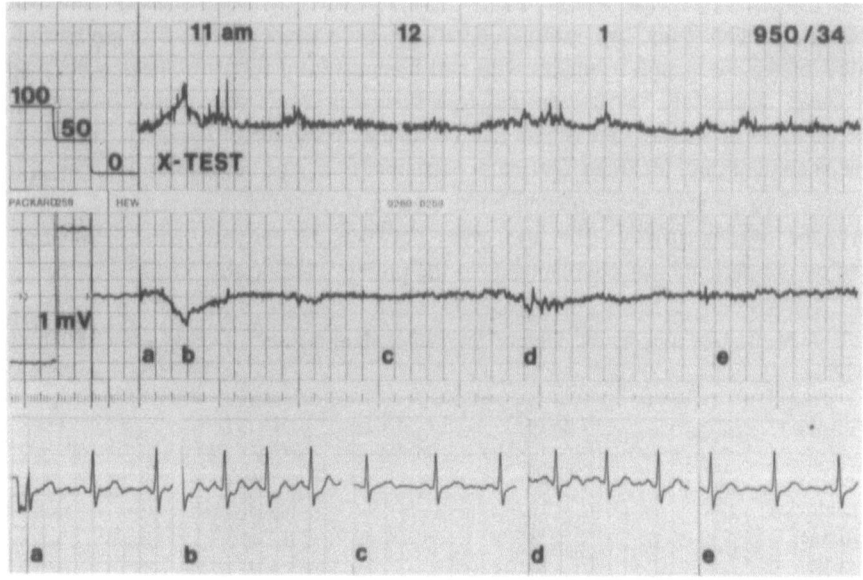

Figure 2. Trend recording of heartrate (top) and ST level (middle) in a patient from group I. The analog output of the play back unit was connected to a stripchart recorder. Note increased heartrate and ST depression during the exercise test at the onset of the recording. During other activities several episodes of ST depression without symptoms occurred.

the Oxford Instruments Medilog II analyser. An experienced technician scanned the tape for rhythm abnormalities and for changes of QRS and ST waveforms, which were then recorded on paper. In addition a trend plot was made of heartrate and the ST level in lead CM_5 throughout the recording period (figure 2). The operator placed one number marker at the PQ segment, just prior to the QRS complex. Another marker was placed approximately 60 msec after the end of QRS. The voltage difference between these two points represented the ST level.

In group I the early version of the Medilog II play back unit was used. The heartrate and ST signals were obtained from analog outputs of the play back unit, passed through a low pass filter and recorded on a stripchart recorder (figure 2). Data from group II were analysed with a later version of the same play back unit. This version averaged the heartrate and ST level at 30 seconds intervals and generated a plot of these average values (figure 3).

ECG strips were made at all instants when changes of the ST level occurred in the trend plots, and when the patient reported any symptoms in the diary. ST segment changes were interpreted as abnormal when a near horizontal ST depression or ST elevation occurred of 0.1 mV or greater compared with the baseline ST level.

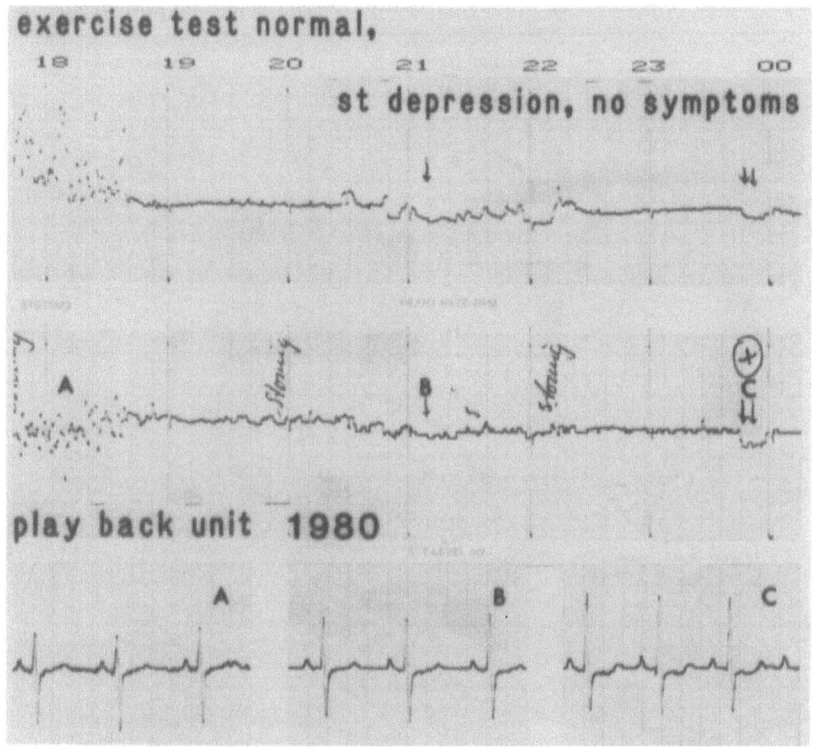

Figure 3. Trend recording of heartrate (top) and ST level (middle) in a patient from group II, with one minute averaging of the measurements. Note noisy signal at the onset of the recording (18–19 o'clock, A). During an episode with reduced heartrate, ST depression occurred in lead CM_5 (C).

Twenty five patients from group I and 12 from group II had an abnormal ST segment response during exercise. In all cases the configuration of the ST changes in lead CM_5 from the ambulatory ECG recording at the time of the stress test were similar to those in the computer processed exercise ECG. The degree of ST depression in lead CM_5 was always greater than in Frank lead X at the same instant (4). The recording system did not cause visible distortions of the ST waveform.

During normal activities 17 patients from group I and 11 from group II had ST depression of 0.1 mV or greater. Twenty five of these patients had an abnormal exercise test, while three had ST changes during ambulatory monitoring and a normal stress test. ST elevation in lead CM_5 was observed in one patient who sustained a myocardial infarction during the recording period and in two patients with a previous anterior wall infarction.

These results agree with other reports (5, 6, 7) as summarized in table 2.

Table 2. Incidence of significant ST-segment changes ($\geqslant 0.1$ mV) by ambulatory electrocardiography (Holter) and exercise testing in the present study and in studies from other centers. Note that most patients had either no ST changes, or changes recorded by both methods. In the other patients exercise testing was more sensitive than ambulatory electrocardiography.

	no ST	Exercise + Holter	Holter	Exercise
Wolf (5)	23	13	5	6
Stern (6)	20	23	2	3
O'Rourke (7)	18	21	7	10
Thorax I	20	17	–	8
Thorax II	16	8	3	4

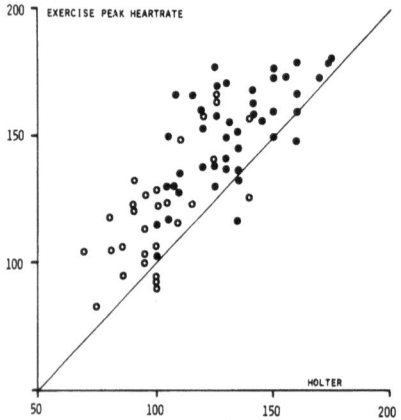

Figure 4. Peak heartrate during the exercise test and during other activities in patients with beta blockers (open circles) and in two other patients. The heartrate levels were measured from the trend recording and checked in the ECG tracings.

In most patients the degree of ST depression during the exercise test exceeded the ST depression in the same ECG lead during other activities (figure 2, table 3). This may be due to the higher heart rate achieved during exercise compared with other activities (figure 4).

The relation between symptoms and ST-changes is summarized in table 4. In both groups only part of the episodes of chest discomfort were accompagnied by ST changes. On the other hand 24 out of 51 episodes with ST depression in group I and 46 out of 56 episodes in group II were asymptomatic.

In the ST trend many episodes of "false positive" ST shifts were observed. These were due to various causes, including ST junction depression at higher heartrate, P wave and QRS changes, premature ventricular complexes, changes in body position, baseline drift and other types of noise.

Ventricular arrhythmias were observed in 24 exercise tests and in 66 ambulatory

Table 3. Distribution of the greatest degree of ST-depression or ST elevation in each patient by ambulatory electrocardiography (vertical) and stress testing (horizontal). 0–4 denote ST changes in mm on the stripchart recorder (1 mV = 10 mm). Note that in most patients ST changes during exercise exceeded those during ambulatory electrocardiography.

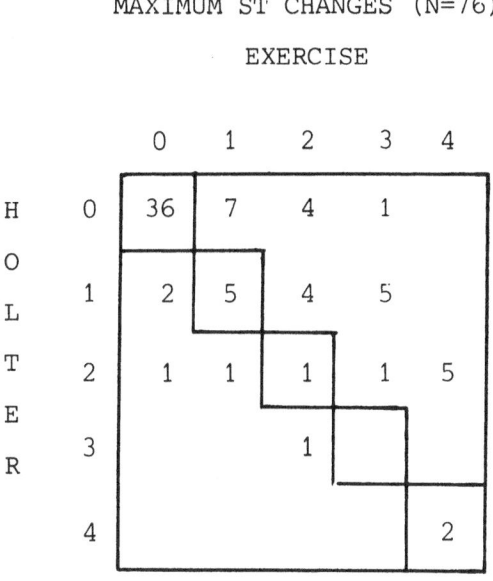

MAXIMUM ST CHANGES (N=76)

EXERCISE

		0	1	2	3	4
H	0	36	7	4	1	
O	1	2	5	4	5	
L T	2	1	1	1	1	5
E	3			1		
R	4					2

Table 4. Incidence of episodes with significant ST changes and/or chest pain in the present study.

ST changes	+	+	–
Chest pain	+	–	+
Angina (n=45; 24 h)	27	24	50
Rehabilitation (n=31; 48 h)	10	46	59

ECG recordings. Usually the arrhythmias were more frequent and more complex in the ambulatory recording as shown in table 5. This difference is most likely related to the duration of the ECG recording which was approximately 20 – 30 minutes during the stress test compared with 24 or 48 hours monitoring (8).

Discussion

The ST segment changes during exercise as recorded by the system for ambulatory monitoring in the present study, were similar to those detected by computer processing of the Frank lead ECG. Thus accurate analysis of ST segment changes by ambulatory monitoring is feasible, provided that a system with adequate

Table 5. Distribution of the highest degree of ventricular arrhythmias in each patient during exercise and during ambulatory electrocardiography in the present study.

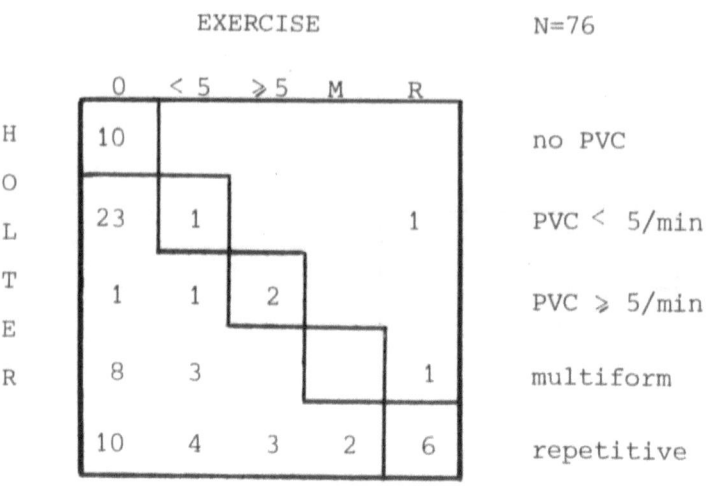

	EXERCISE					N=76
	0	< 5	≥ 5	M	R	
H	10					no PVC
O						
L	23	1			1	PVC < 5/min
T	1	1	2			PVC ≥ 5/min
E						
R	8	3			1	multiform
	10	4	3	2	6	repetitive

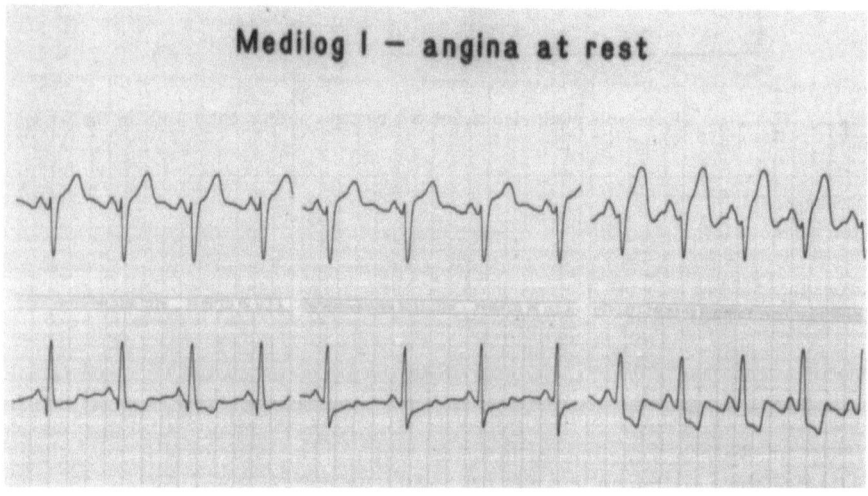

Medilog I — angina at rest

Figure 5. Gross ST segment change during an episode of chest pain in a patient with Prinzmetal angina. This recording was made with a system which is not designed for correct reproduction of the ECG waveform.

frequency response is used (1, 2, 5–7). In some patients large ST changes may be observed occasionally, even when a system is used which is clearly not designed for this purpose (figure 5). Such gross ST changes probably indicate myocardial ischemia when they occur during an episode of chest pain. However, routine use of such systems for ST segment analysis should be avoided, in order to prevent false positive as well as false negative findings. Data from the present study support earlier reports (8) that ambulatory electrocardiography gives a greater yield of rhythm disturbances than stress testing. On the other hand exercise testing remains the method of choice for detection of myocardial ischemia in patients with chest pain. ST changes during exercise in the present study appeared more frequently and were often greater than during ambulatory monitoring, even when the same lead and the same recording system were used in both conditions. This is probably related to the greater level of work achieved as reflected by higher heartrates during the exercise test (figure 4). Greater ST changes may be achieved during monitoring if the patient is instructed to perform strenuous exercise during the monitoring period. However, such unsupervised stress testing carries increased risk for complications including sudden death in patients with coronary disease (9, 10). On the other hand, ambulatory electrocardiography may be more sensitive than stress testing for detection of episodes of myocardial ischemia which are not related to increased oxygen demand but to decreased coronary blood flow caused by increased vasomotor activity.

A disadvantage of ambulatory monitoring is the limitation to 2 ECG leads. The majority of cases with ST depression during exercise induced myocardial ischemia can be detected in lead CM_5 (11). However, ST changes may only appear in other leads (12), in particular in patients with a previous myocardial infarction and in patients with chest pain due to enhanced vasomotor activity of the coronary arteries. Thus the absence of significant ST segment changes during episodes of chest pain does not exclude that such episodes are related to myocardial ischemia. In particular, the large amount of such episodes in the patients from the rehabilitation program is disturbing. (table 4). Furthermore it should be realized that an exercise test provides additional information which is of equal diagnostic and prognostic significance as the ECG: in particular determination of exercise tolerance and the hemodynamic response to stress. At present, limited data is available on the relation between ST segment changes during ambulatory monitoring and the presence or absence of coronary artery disease. In our series, no comparison with coronary arteriography was done. Results from three other centers (6, 7, 13) indicate that the sensitivity and specificity for detection of coronary artery disease may be similar for ambulatory electrocardiography and stress testing, provided that the same criteria are used for interpretation of the ECG. Such results will depend heavily on the selection of patients in a particular study, and on the equipment employed. In our experience, exercise testing is likely to be more sensitive in patients with classical angina, while ambulatory electrocardiography may be of advantage in variant angina.

In the present study ST segment depression was interpreted as a sign of myocardial ischemia. ST elevation during an episode of chest pain occurred in one patient only. In addition ST elevation was observed in patients with a previous anterior wall infarction. This is most likely due to the presence of a large area with scan tissue, or even an aneurysm of the left ventricle (14). In many patients alterations of the T wave, including T inversion were observed during ambulatory monitoring. These alterations were not related to symptomas, and should not be regarded as a sign of myocardial ischemia.

A recording of the trends of heartrate and the ST level in our experience contributes to the detection of episodes with ST segment changes. However, many other factors may cause a shift of the ST trend. Thus it is mandatory to check the original ECG in all instances when a shift in the ST trend is observed. "False" ST shifts were most often due to frequent premature beats, noise and changes of body position.

At present the methods employed for measurement of the ST segment in ambulatory monitoring are rather simple. More reliable methods have been developed for computer processing of exercise electrocardiograms (15). Application of such methods in ambulatory electrocardiography is limited by the high sample rate required when a tape is played back at e.g. 60x normal speed. When faster processors become available, processing of ambulatory ECGs for ST (and QRS) analysis in the near future should include: simultaneous analysis of 2 or more ECG leads; detection of premature beats as well as beats with excessive noise levels; averaging of the dominant type of QRS complex; determination of the proper onset and end of QRS in the averaged signal; and measurement of both ST-amplitude and ST-slope, possibly in relation to heartrate at each instant (15). In addition measurements from the QRS complex may be employed to estimate changes in left ventricular volume. However, present data on the significance of such changes during exercise are conflicting (11).

It is concluded that ambulatory ST segment monitoring is feasible and reliable when proper equipment is employed. Nevertheless exercise testing remains the method of choice for detection of myocardial ischemia in patients with chest pain. Ambulatory ST segment monitoring may be indicated a) in patients with chest pain and a normal exercise test, in particular when the symptoms are not related to physical stress; b) in patients with symptoms at rest or during specific activities; c) in patients who are unable to exercise. Finally, ambulatory ST segment monitoring may be used to determine the number of episodes of myocardial ischemia in a patient with known coronary disease, for example in the evaluation of the efficacy of drug treatment.

Acknowledgements

The author acknowledges the contributions of Ton Boehmer MD, Phons Fels MD, Inge Linstra and Jos de Laat who collected the data for the present study. The ambulatory ECG recordings were analysed by Angela Peterse and Suze Schendeling, Cardiolab – Rotterdam. Flora ten Cate and Hanneke van Meurs assisted the exercise tests. The manuscript was prepared, with the aid of Anneke Wagenaar.

References

1. Bragg-Remschel D.A. 1981. New methods to evaluate the frequency response and ST segment reproducibility of ambulatory ECG systems. Computers in Cardiology, in press.
2. Balasubramanian V, Lahiri A, Green HL, Stott FD, Raftery EB. 1980. Br Heart J 44: 419–25.
3. Vinke RVM, Engelse WAH, Hooghoudt T, Mey S, Simoons ML, Top P, Zeelenberg C. 1977. Implementation and clinical evaluation of computer assisted analysis of exercise ECG. In: Computers in Cardiology. Santa Barbara, Calif, IEEE Computer Society, p. 345.
4. Hornsten TR, Bruce RA. 1969. Computed ST forces of Frank and bipolar exercise electrocardiograms. Am. Heart J. 78: 346–357.
5. Wolf E, Tzivoni D, Stern S. 1974. Comparison of exercise tests and 24-hour ambulatory electrocardiographic monitoring in detection of ST-T changes. Br Heart H 36: 93.
6. Stern S. 1978. Ambulatory ECG-monitoring. Year Book Medical Publishers Inc., Chicago.
7. O'Rourke R, Crawford MH. 1978. The value of ambulatory electrocardiographic monitoring for detection of ischemic heart disease. Advances in heart disease. Mason DT, Ed. Green and Shaffon, New York.
8. Ryan M, Lown B, Horn H. 1975. Comparison of ventricular ectopic activity during 24 hour monitoring and exercise testing in patients with coronary heart disease. New Eng. J. Med. 292: 224–229.
9. Irving JB, Bruce RA. 1977. Exertional hypotension and postexertional ventricular fibrillation in stress testing. Amer J Cardiol. 39: 849.
10. Scherer D, Kaltenbach M. 1979. Haufigkeit lebensbedrohlicher Komplikationen bei ergometrischen Belastungsuntersuchungen. Dtsch. med. Wschr. 104: 1161–1175.
11. Simoons ML, Block P. 1981. Toward the optimal lead system and optimal criteria for exercise electrocardiography. Amer J Cardiol 47: 1366–1374.
12. Chaitman BR, Waters DD, Theroux P, Hanson JS. 1981. S-T segment elevation and coronary spasm in response to exercise. Amer. J Cardiol. 47: 1350–1358.
13. Kukes SH, Pichard A, Meller J, Gorlin R, Herman MV, Kupersmith J. 1980. Use of the ambulatory ECG to diagnose coronary artery disease. J. Electrocardiol. 13: 341–346.
14. Simoons ML, Pool J, Brand M v/d, Hugenholtz RG, 1978. Quantitative analysis of exercise electrocardiograms. Adv. Cardiol. vol. 21, pp. 326–329.
15. Simoons ML, Hugenholtz PG, Ascoop CA, Distelbrink CA, Land PA de, Vinke RVM. 1981. Quantitation of exercise electrocardiography. Circulation 63, 3: 471–475.

CONTINUOUS BLOOD PRESSURE MEASUREMENT

PETER SLEIGHT, M.D., F.R.C.P.

Cuff blood pressure measurement has changed very little since the beginning of this century and has provided an immense amount of valuable data on outcome and risk. Restrictions of the technique make it of limited value in sleep, exercise or at work, although there are now devices which inflate and deflate automatically. Perhaps the biggest problem is the alerting or defence reaction which is engendered by the observer or even by the cuff inflation with automatic devices. For this reason there have been many attempts to develop systems which track blood pressure non invasively. We have used the measurement of pulse wave velocity to follow beat to beat changes in pressure (1). This and similar systems have not so far proved adequate for ambulatory use, and all indirect systems have severe problems with calibration and validation.

We have therefore preferred to concentrate on direct intra arterial measurements and have refined the method originally developed in the late Sir George Pickering's Department in Oxford by Bevan, Honour and Stott (2). The first device was ingenious but relatively crude. It recorded pressure by a strain gauge onto a tiny strip of photosensitive paper moved slowly by a watch mechanism. It was therefore only possible to record broad changes in pressure. Beat to beat analysis was not possible and there was no record of the ECG. The brachial artery cannula was flushed by saline pressurised by butane gas and a rubber diaphragm. The whole device was somewhat temperamental. The most important step was to record the data on magnetic tape using the Oxford Instruments Medilog recorder (again based on an invention by Stott). With this one could then measure many more variables – ECG, eye movement, respiration, locomotion etc. Automatic analysis of the data was also possible. With this device we were able to show the normal variability of blood pressure under various conditions of work or leisure including sleep and dreams (4), exercise (3), coitus (5), defaecation and micturition (6), cigarette smoking (7), car driving (8), etc.

Methods

We now use the following technique: using careful sterile precautions a needle is inserted in the brachial artery about 3 centimetres above the elbow crease, under local anaesthesia. Through this is threaded a fine wire and the needle is withdrawn. A short polythene catheter (0.6 mm i.d.) is threaded over the wire and the latter is withdrawn. In skilled hands the procedure is painless and atraumatic; only the anterior wall of the artery is punctured. The polythene cannula is then connected by one metre of fine polythene tube to a pressure gauge/perfusion system worn at heart level in a pouch suspended round the neck. The transducer is an Akers semiconductor strain gauge. The perfusion system is now more reliable and uses a miniature roller pump powered by hearing aid batteries. This perfuses about 1 ml/h of sterile water and heparin (100 μ/ml) down the brachial artery cannula.

Complications

Over the last 12 years we have carried out several hundred such procedures and had only 3 serious complications. These 3 median nerve palsies were reported by Littler (9). We are not entirely sure of the mechanism in these 3 cases but we then changed our technique in two ways and have not had any further problems over the last few years.

We first avoided the temptation to puncture the artery at the elbow crease where it is most easily felt. In this location the nerve and artery are tightly constrained by the biceps aponeurosis and the nerve is therefore particularly vulnerable to pressure from any haematoma. Second – and I personally feel this is very important – we avoid too heavy pressure on the site of withdrawal of the cannula after the study. In one case of ours the electroneurogram suggested that the lesion was above the level of the puncture site. Heavy and prolonged pressure on nerves is known to produce ischaemic necrosis.

We have had no instance of arterial thrombosis or systemic infection; we exclude patients with lesions which make them at risk of bacterial endocarditis. There is occasionally a troublesome haematoma, especially in elderly subjects with sclerotic arteries. The catheter is usually well tolerated. Our usual procedure is to record for 24 hours and then remove the cannula. In a few cases we have left the system in for 48 hours. Raftery's group at Northwick Park Hospital who use the same technique have left the cannula in for up to 4 days without serious problems. In one patient where there was a strong clinical need (tetanus with autonomic "storms") we have left the cannula in for 3 weeks.

We are careful to obtain informed consent from the subjects. In many cases we have repeated the procedure in the same person before and after treatment. The procedure is invasive and potentially hazardous, I have therefore restricted the arterial puncture procedure to myself and usually not more than one other

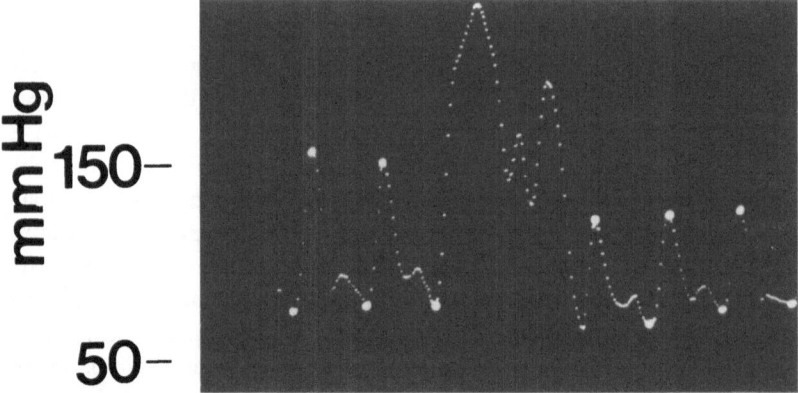

Figure 1. Shows oscilloscope playback to the person editing the tape. The brightened up points represent the systolic and diastolic pressures stored by the computer; the movement artefact in the middle has been edited out.

senior person in my department at any time. It is *not* a procedure to be handed down from one research fellow to the next. Very great care is necessary when flushing or calibrating the system. It also depends very heavily on skilled and experienced servicing of the pressure/perfusion unit. There is also a big investment in computer skills to obtain reliable and artefact free data. I am very happy to acknowledge the contribution of our engineer Mr. J. Johnston, who deserves most of the credit for our present trouble free system.

Mr. Johnston has developed a sophisticated analysis system (10). The tape is digitised (100 Hz) and is played onto the disk of a Data General Eclipse S200 mini-computer at 25 times speed to that the 24 hour record is captured in about one hour. An observer can scan the quality of the record from the disk on an oscilloscope which displays 3 or 5 pulses at a time at up to 60 times real time. Normally these pulses oscillate up and down the screen in a smooth fashion as the blood pressure rises and falls. Movement and artefact or other interference is seen as a sudden unnatural jerk in the display. The operator then scans back the tape slowly in real time and edits out any bogus pulses by pressing a typewriter key.

He also "marks" any pulses which appear to be damped (either from a kink in the catheter or tubing or because of partial occlusion of the catheter against the arterial wall). The computer keeps count of these edited or "marked" pulses and prints out a display of when these occurred and what percentage of beats at that time have been edited. In this way the quality of the original data can be seen on the final record. (fig. 2)

The computer calculates the systolic, diastolic and integrated mean arterial pressures and pulse interval. The points it has taken for systole and diastole are brightened up in the operators display screen so that he can check what has been recorded.

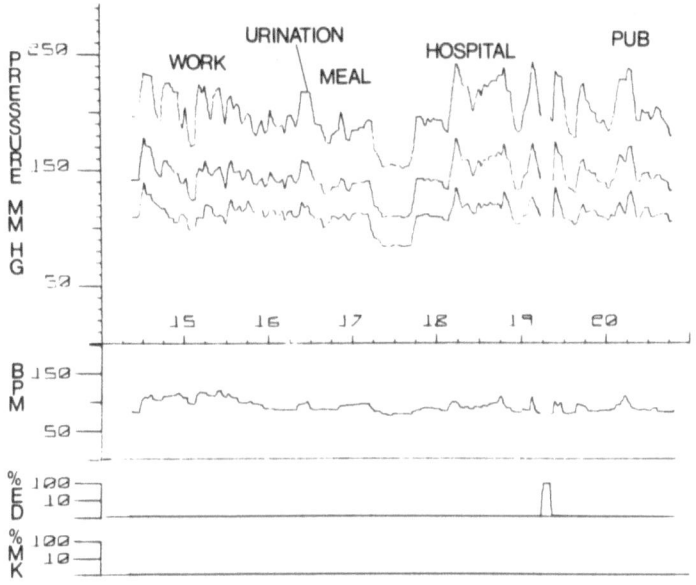

Figure 2. A 6 hour print out of 2 minutes means of systolic and diastolic and computed mean pressures and heart rate (BPM). A small portion was at the time of the evening calibration at 1915 hours and was edited out (%Ed). No traces were considered damped (%MK). The variability is clearly seen. Note the rise in pressure when attending hospital for the calibration.

The machine stores averages and standard deviation of each 2 minutes of all these variables and plots this as a 24 hour or expanded 6 hour chart on A4 paper suitable for the patients' records. It also prints out hourly means and S.D. and can produce histograms of these and the total data.

Advantages of Direct Arterial Continuous Ambulatory Records

We make these recordings for several purposes.

First where there is a doubt about the readings obtained by the cuff technique. This is not a rare problem. We are all familiar with the patient who defies control of blood pressure despite powerful and multiple drug regimes, yet appears to suffer little or no target organ damage. Some years ago we culled our hypertension clinic records and picked out such individuals. We measured their true intra-arterial record on treatment and compared this with their averaged cuff pressures. There was a large discrepancy as a result of falsely high cuff readings. This was not due to an artefact of the cuff method (e.g. due to fat arms) but to an exaggerated defence reaction in the face of doctors. A control group of more conventional hypertensives gave much better agreement between cuff and intraarterial readings (11).

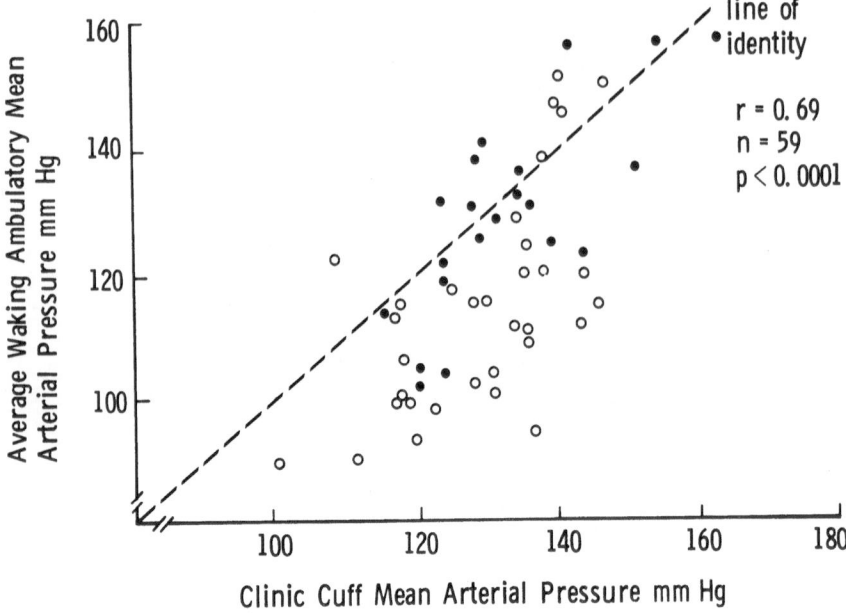

Figure 3. Comparison of intra-arterial pressures away from hospital (including activity) and the "resting" cuff pressures at clinic attendance. Open circles show subjects free from target organ damage (from Floras et al, 13 with permission).

In a later study of untreated subjects recruited for a trial of mild to moderate hypertension we were surprised to find just how common this problem might be. As a result of at least 3 cuff blood pressure readings over 140/90 mm Hg direct ambulatory records were done on 59 patients. In no less than 20 subjects the average awake mean arterial pressure was found to be less than 108 mm Hg equivalent to 140/90) and in many cases was considerably less (12).

Another important finding was that there was no easy or obvious clinical distinction (pulse rate, reaction to mental arithmetic, plasma catecholamines) between those subjects whose cuff blood pressure was an accurate estimate of their true arterial pressure and those where the cuff pressures were much higher. We do not think that artefacts of measurement were responsible for we compared careful simultaneous cuff and arterial pressures in many of these subjects; we found cuff systolic pressure accurately recorded the true systolic pressure, but diastolic pressure was over estimated by the cuff, whether 4th or 5th phase was taken.

We did find (like Sokolow and his colleagues (13) using home blood pressure measurement) that those with good agreement between clinic cuff and direct ambulatory blood pressures had more target organ damage (12).

With increasing evidence in favour of the treatment of relatively mild hypertension it is very important to be sure of the accuracy of our assessment. It is not desirable or practicable to carry out direct recording of arterial pressure but it is likely that home blood pressure measurement either by the patient or spouse or by some well validated method such as the Remmler system used by Sokolow will help resolve this problem.

As well as determining whether the individual has true hypertension which needs treatment we also use the method to obtain data for the patient which may be acceptable to insurance companies who have refused or loaded life insurance premiums because of alleged hypertension. Home blood pressure records from patient or spouse cuff techniques are obviously not applicable here!

A third important use for the technique is in the evaluation of the efficacy and duration of action of drugs. The intraarterial ambulatory record differs surprisingly little in any individual from day to day, provided that similar activities are carried out on each day.

Gould and his colleagues in Northwick Park have shown that the technique removes the "placebo" effect which so bedevils clinical trials (14). They carried out 3 separate intra arterial studies on each subject who was randomly allocated to no tablet, placebo, or active drug.

A "placebo" fall in pressure was seen with the placebo tablet when *cuff* measurements were taken and compared with no tablet; the intra arterial traces under these conditions showed no significant difference.

In a recent trial of 4 different beta adrenoceptor blocking agents (Atenolol, long acting Propranolol, Metoprolol and Pindolol,) given on a once daily regime we found that the shorter half life Metropolol needed to be given twice daily for effective 24 hour control, or as a slow release preparation. Pindolol which has considerable partial agonist activity (sometimes called ISA) differed in that the sleeping pulse rate was actually higher on treatment than off; this is presumably because the P.A.A. became dominant at a time when the natural sympathetic drive is reduced. The blood pressure at night was also not reduced by Pindolol given in a once daily morning dose.

A fourth use of the technique is to evaluate causes of inexplicable "turns" when other investigations have failed; one may find falls in blood pressure due to autonomic disturbances which have not been revealed by routine methods.

Finally the method is of great value in the investigation of the aetiology and mechanism of so called essential hypertension, when it is necessary to correlate other measures (e.g. of baroreflex control, plasma catecholamines or of salt intake) with a subject's arterial pressure. We have seen that we may be considerably misled if we rely only on cuff methods which are muddled by the defence reaction.

References

1. Gribbin B, Steptoe A, Sleight P. Pulse wave velocity as a measurement of blood pressure change. Psychophysiology 1976; 13: 86–90.
2. Bevan AT, Honour AJ, Stott FD. Direct arterial pressure recording in unrestricted man. Clin Sci 1969; 36: 329–44.
3. Littler WA, Honour AJ, Sleight P, Stott FD. Continuous recording of direct arterial pressure and electrocardiogram in unrestricted man. Br Med J 1972; iii: 76–78.

4. Bristow JD, Honour AJ, Pickering TG, Sleight P. Cardiovascular and respiratory changes during sleep in normal and hypertensive subjects. Cardiovasc Res 1969; 3: 476–485.

5. Littler WA, Honour AJ, Sleight P. Direct arterial pressure, heart rate and electrocardiogram during human coitus. J Reproduct Fertil 1974; 40: 321–331.

6. Littler WA, Honour AJ, Sleight P. Direct Arterial pressure, pulse rate and electrocardiogram during micturition and defaecation in unrestricted man. Amer Heart J 1874; 88: 205–210.

7. Cellina GU, Honour AJ, Littler WA. Direct arterial pressure, heart rate and electrocardiogram during cigarette smoking in unrestricted patients. Amer Heart J 1975; 89: 18–25.

8. Littler WA, Honour AJ, Sleight P. Direct arterial pressure and electrocardiogram during motor car driving. Brit Med J 1973; 2: 273–277.

9. Littler WA. Median nerve palsy; a complication of brachial artery cannulation. Post grad Med J 1976; 52 (supp 7): 110–111.

10. Sleight P, Jones JV, Floras J. Automatic analysis of continuous intra-arterial blood pressure recordings. Index: blood pressure variability (Clement DL ed) Lancaster, MTP press, 1979; 55–60.

11. Littler WA, Honour AJ, Pugsley DJ, Sleight P. Continuous recording of direct arterial pressure in unrestricted patients: its role in the diagnosis and management of high blood pressure. Circulation 1975; 51: 1101–106.

12. Floras JS, Hassan MO, Sever P, Jones JV, Osikowska B, Sleight P. Cuff and ambulatory blood pressure in subjects with essential hypertension. Lancet July 1981; 107–109.

13. Sokolow M, Werdegar D, Kain HK, Hinman AT. Relationship between blood pressure measured casually and by portable recorders and severity of complications in essential hypertension. Circulation 1966; 34: 279–289.

14. Gould BA, Mann S, Altman D, Raftery EB. Can placebo therapy in clinical trials really influence the blood pressure. Clin Sci 1981. In press.

APPLICATION OF HOLTER ELECTROCARDIOGRAPHY TO PHYSIOLOGICAL MEASUREMENTS IN MAN

K. BACHMANN

Different technical approaches to laboratory-remote recording of cardiovascular parameters are presently available: transmission by radio and phone on the one hand and storage telemetry using tape- or solid-state-recording on the other. Today's most applied method of "medical telecommunication" is tape-recording and the signal measured routinely has always been the electrocardiogram (Fig. 1).

Looking back in history we find that EINTHOVEN developed his télécardiogramme in 1906 to bridge the distance between hospital and laboratory to record the electrocardiogram for diagnostic purposes. When after World War II, HOLTER started to develop ECG-telemetry his intention was to have a method of measuring everyday cardiovascular stress using heart rate samples as an indicator. This explains why HOLTER in 1949 entitled his first publication on this subject "remote-recording of physiological data by radio". Recording of the R-R-interval presented the least technical difficulty. Heart rate profile was easily obtained, ups and downs were no problem for interpretation. Up to now heart rate has been used as an indicator of environmental hemodynamic stress and cardiovascular response to it. In the second stage of technical advance with the development of light-weight patient-borne devices the "HOLTER Monitor Test" (CORDAY et al. 1965. HOLTER, 1961, 1963, 1972) was used primarily for diagnostic and prognostic purposes in patients with arrhythmias. With further technical refinement and introduction of frequency-modulated tape-recording application of HOLTER monitoring has nowadays been extended to patients with coronary heart disease.

With regard to the widespread use of HOLTER electrocardiography we may ask the question: how sensitive is this method in evaluating the physiological stress imposed on the cardiovascular system? This is linked with the further question: how closely do changes in heart rate correlate with physical activity and emotional stress in terms of pressure and rate-pressure-product. Thus the question turns out to be a physiological rather than a methodological one. During laboratory dynamic exercise testing the rise in heart rate is linear correlated to the increase in oxygen consumption. This is the reason why HOLTER electrocardiography for recording heart rate is "the most frequently employed measure of physical effort" (BASSEY, FENTEM 1980).

Long-term ambulatory
electrocardiography   FdB

106

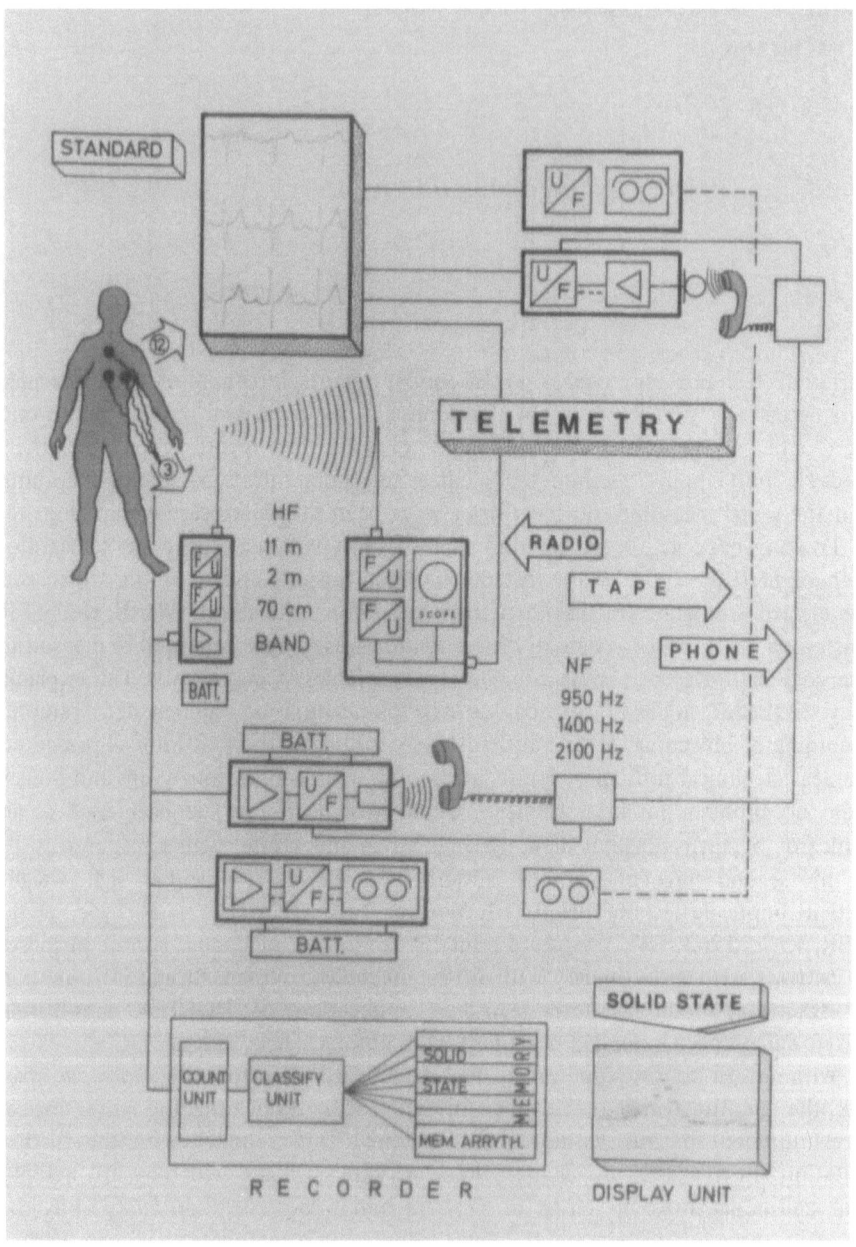

Figure 1. Schematic drawing of technology for laboratory-remote recording of cardiovascular parameters: transmission by radio and phone, storage-telemetry by tape- and solid-state-recording.

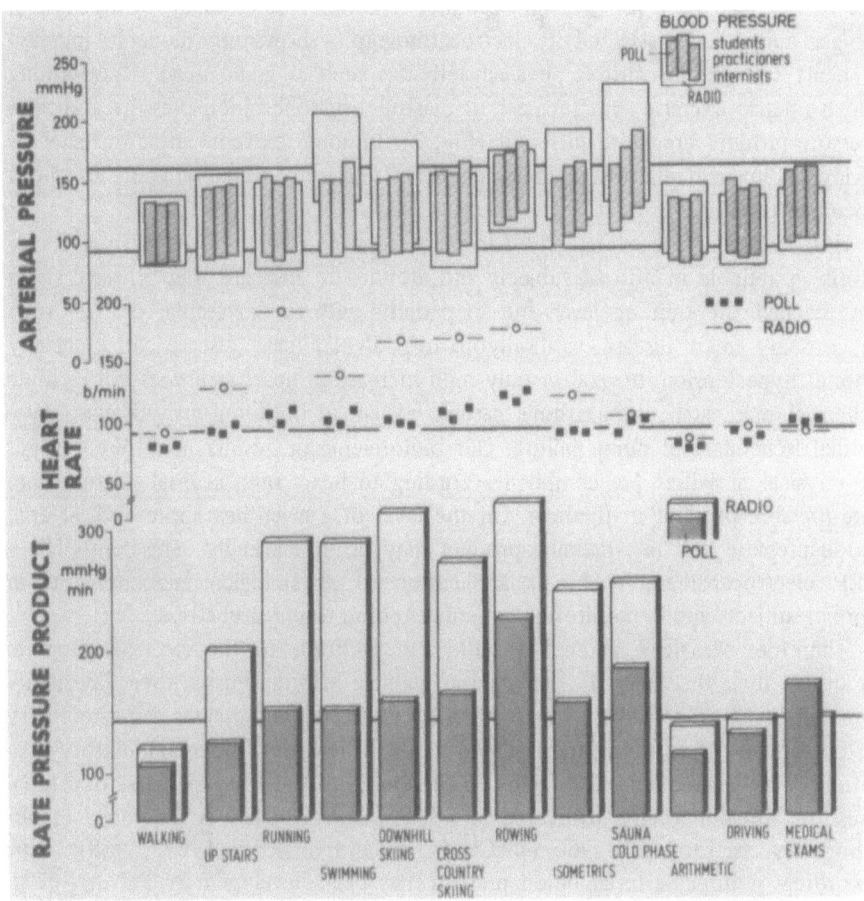

Figure 2. Comparison of a questionnaire with radiotelemetric data. There are great differences between estimats and results of radiotelemtric measurements in normal subjects exposed to everyday stress, sport and extreme situations. Furthermore it becomes appearent that the rise in heart rate ist not correlated neither with arterial pressure nor rate-pressure-product.

In order to evaluate the application of the HOLTER electrocardiography to physiological measurements we performed ratiotelemetry of the electrocardiogram and of direct continuous blood pressure measurements in the arterial system simultaneously. From the results of these physiological data which differ markedly from a questionnaire one surely must conclude that heart rate profile is reliable during dynamic and emotional stress only (Fig. 2). HOLTER electrocardiography may mislead completely in the evaluation of everyday hemodynamic stress in terms of pre-load and after-load and in indicating myocardial oxygen demand. This is especially true during isometric stress with excessive increase of both systolic and diastolic blood pressure. In comparing different physical activities there is no correlation between the increment of systolic and diastolic blood pressure and the rise of heart rate and rate-pressure-product as a major determinant of myocardial oxygen demand. Thus HOLTER electrocardiography shows only moderate increase in heart rate during various physical activities such as going upstairs, swimming and isometric exercise, but increase in diastolic, systolic blood pressure and rate-pressure-product are quite different (Fig. 2). In some extreme situations such as diving an inverse relationship between heart rate and arterial pressure has been documented (Fig. 3).

HOLTER electrocardiography for physiological studies using the heart rate profile is reliable in normal subjects and athletes to indicate that physical stress has reached the training level. But in patients with cardiovascular diseases such as coronary heart disease, cardiomyopathy, valvular heart disease and especially arterial hypertension, normal or only mild increase in heart rate does not exclude potential risk, such as hazardous cardiac over-load initiating arrhythmias, myocardial ischemia and pump failure. Our radiotelemetric results in different types of physical activities are compiled according to heart rate, arterial pressure and rate-pressure-product in figure 4. On the level of a given heart rate both arterial blood pressure and rate-pressure-product may differ markedly. This limits HOLTER electrocardiography in its application to physiological measurements in normal subjects and in monitoring patients exposed to physical stress.

Therefore we need parameters either in addition to the electrocardiogram or others than the ECG. To get a more realistic information on everyday hemodynamic stress, especially in patients with cardiovascular diseases, we should try to perform the measurements available in the laboratory under ambulatory conditions. At the moment additionally to the electrocardiogram telemetry of arterial pressure and pulmonary artery pressure is available which was developed in our laboratory as early as 1966 (BACHMANN and THEBIS 1967, 1968). Tape recording of direct arterial blood pressure has been developed by BEVAN et al. 1969 and improved by LITTLER et al. (1972). Pulmonary artery pressure indicates pre-load, arterial pressure after-load and the calculated rate-pressure-product reflects myocardial oxygen demand. What we cannot record is cardiac output, left ventricular volumes and vascular resistance. By adding HOLTER electrocardiography to radiotransmission of direct pressure measurements in the arterial system and pulmonary artery we get a broad information about the cardiovascular performance in fully ambulatory patients.

It should be emphasized that this extension of laboratory remote recording technique by telemetry is for research purposes primarily but not exclusively. Basically, we have the technical option of performing telemetry of various cardiovascular parameters by tape-recording. It makes no difference whether the frequency-modulated or pulse-code-modulated signals are taken on tape or transmitted by radio. But for monitoring blood pressure with the ballon-tipped SWAN-GANZ catheter in the pulmonary artery and a microcatheter in the femoral or brachial artery simultaneously we recommend continuous monitoring of the patient on a scope and guidance by medical staff. With this precaution no serious complications have occurred in more than 2 500 invasive examinations outside

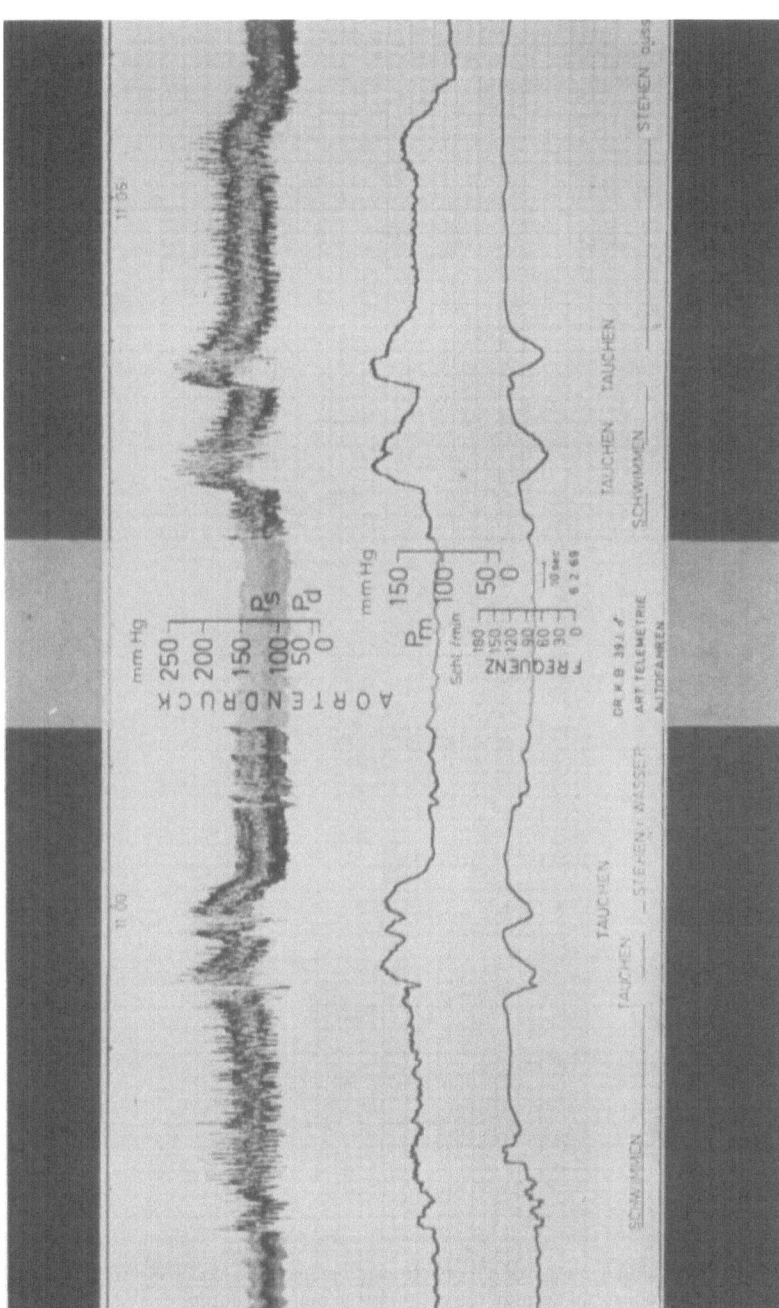

Figure 3. Radiotransmission of direct continuous arterial blood pressure measurements during swimming (Schwimmen) and diving (Tauchen) in a 39-year old healthy subject. During diving there is an inverse relationship between arterial blood pressure and heart rate. Arterial blood pressure increases to a maximum of 250/160 mm Hg while heart rate decreases down to 50 b/min (self-test, February 6 th 1969).

110

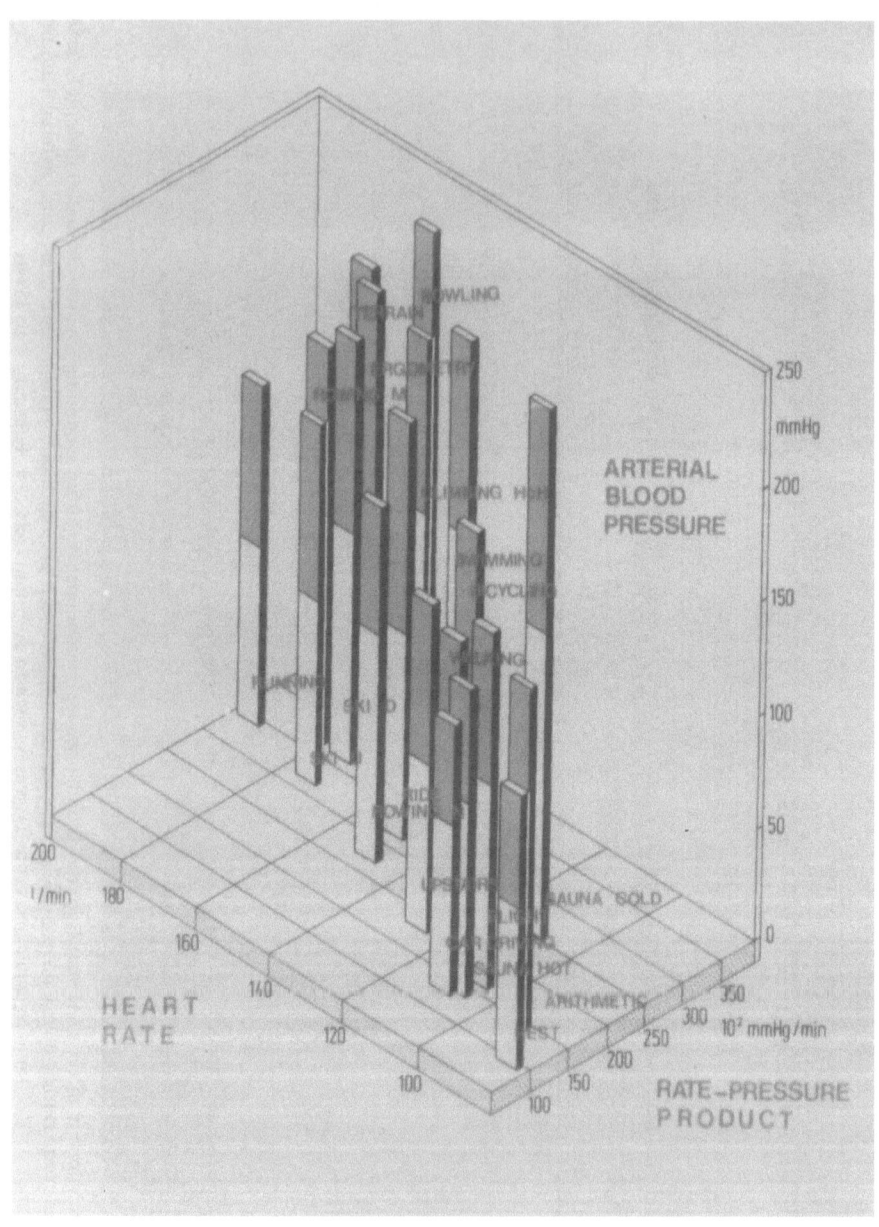

Figure 4. Results of radiotelemetry of the electrocardiogram, the arterial pressure and calculated pressure-rate-product in normotensive subjects monitored during everyday activites and sports.

the hospital since 1966. More than 200 examinations were performed in patients older than 60 years with measuring periods of 6 to 8 hours as an average. In doing so in outpatients we can analyse heart rate, electrical instability of the myocardium, myocardial ischemia and left ventricular performance in patients exposed to physical activity and mental stress during everyday activities, sports and occupational life and even in those extreme situations which cannot be simulated in the laboratory (BACHMANN et al. 1971, 1976, 1978). Furthermore, HOLTER electrocardiography in combination with recording of direct oressure measurements is a valuable method for the evaluation of medical treatment in complete ambulatory patients. Only a few of the many applications can be given as example of how combined telemetry covers a great variety of situations which cannot be simulated in the laboratory. Moreover, such recordings demonstrate both the possibilities and limitations of HOLTER electrocardiography in physiological measurements.

The hemodynamic reflection of physical activity and emotional stress on the cardiovascular system is of special interest in patients with coronary heart disease, in whom we performed radiotelemetry of the electrocardiogram, of pulmonary artery pressure and arterial pressure during walking in the terrain, in the sauna bath, driving a car and during exposure to high altitude hypoxemia (BACHMANN et al. 1971, 1976, 1978). Walking in the terrain provokes in a severely ill group of 15 coronary patients an increase in arterial pressure from 132/75 mm Hg to 176/85 mm Hg with rise in heart rate from 83 to 151 b/min. There is a concomitant increase of pulmonary artery pressure from 24/12 mm Hg to 52/26 mm Hg. Angina is preceded by a sharp rise in both systolic and diastolic pulmonary artery blood pressure and ST-segment depression. Nitrates such as Isosorbiddinitrate given as a single dose of 10 mg s.l. cause a markedly drop in both pulmonary artery and arterial pressure (Fig. 5, Table 1).

The same measurements were performed in coronary patients during driving a car. There is only a moderate increase in heart rate, arterial pressure and pulmonary artery pressure (Table 1). The arterial pressure increases from 134/71 mm Hg to 155/82 mm Hg with rise in heart rate from 67 to 83 b/min. Pulmonary artery pressure increases from 19/7 mm Hg to 25/10 mm Hg. The rate-pressure-product stays in the normal range and coronary insufficiency is far from being provoked by driving, the vasospastic and vasotonic type excluded. When the patient repeats driving under ISDN-medication there is a marked fall in arterial pressure down to 122/72 mm Hg. Pulmonary artery pressure comes down to 15/4 mm Hg. Normally this reaction which includes the potential risk of arterial hypotension is prevented either by the supine position in the laboratory or by physical activity during everyday life. In this special situation of sitting and being exposed to mental stress only the nitrate-induced venous pooling is not counteracted (Fig. 6).

The potential risk of arterial hypotension becomes obvious in our measurements in extreme situations such as being with coronary patients at a non-pressurized aircraft at altitudes between 10 000 and 19 000 feet. Those physicians who are familiar with this condition would consider it a risk to expose coronary patients with severe three-vessel disease and left ventricular disfunction due to myocardial

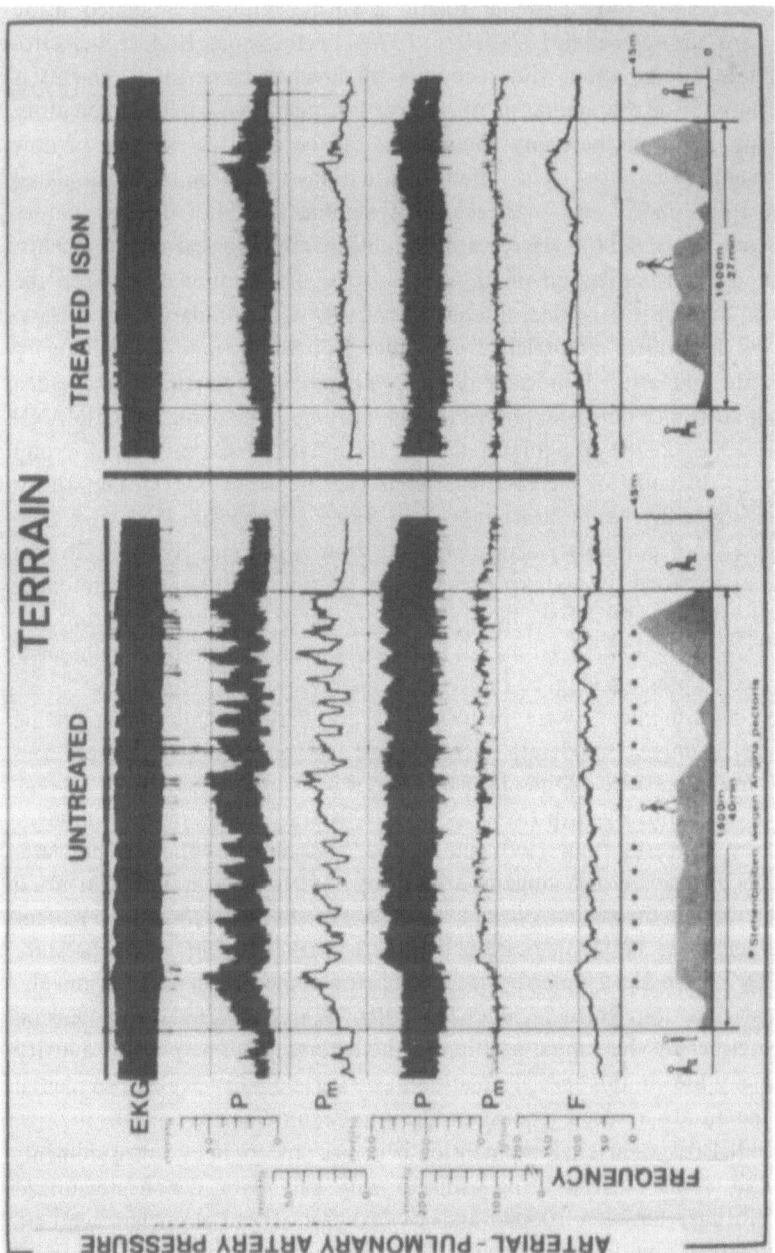

Figure 5. Radiotelemetry of the electrocardiogram and continuous blood pressure measurements in a 51-year old patient with severe coronary heart disease during walking in the terrain before and after s.l. intake of 10 mg of Isosorbiddinitrate.

Table 1. Results of radiotelemetry of direct continuous blood pressure measurements in the arterial system and the pulmonary artery in patients with angiographically documented coronary hwart disease exposed to physical activity in the terrain and mental stress during driving a car.

| | ARTERIAL PRESSURE mm Hg | | | PULMONARY ARTERY PRESSURE mm Hg | | | HEARTRATE b/min |
	systolic	diastolic	mean	systolic	diastolic	mean	
n = 9							
Rest	131,8 ± 17,9	74,3 ± 9,0	96,4 ± 12,0	23,0 ± 4,4	10,4 ± 2,6	16,6 ± 2,6	81,3 ± 12,5
Terrain before	161,4 ± 24,19	81,7 ± 13,3	112,0 ± 17,0	47,4 ± 5,4	22,0 ± 5,3	35,3 ± 5,3	144,4 ± 25,6
Terrain after s.l. 10 mg ISDN	146,4 ± 25,8**	74,1 ± 14,3**	101,6 ± 17,9**	44,1 ± 5,8	20,7 ± 4,4	31,2 ± 4,9*	160,3 ± 13,4*
n = 5							
Rest	134 ± 19,2	71 ± 9,4	93,8 ± 8,8	19,2 ± 3,6	7,2 ± 2,8	12,0 ± 2,4	66,8 ± 8,0
Driving before	155,4 ± 23,2	81,8 ± 7,5	110 ± 13,7	25,2 ± 7,4	10,2 ± 3,1	16,2 ± 5,5	83,4 ± 4,5
Driving after s.l. 10 mg ISDN	121,6 ± 27,6***	72,4 ± 8,7**	88,8 ± 13,9***	15,0 ± 2,1**	4,0 ± 1,1	9,8 ± 1,9*	70,2 ± 39,7

*** p = 0,001
** p = 0,01
* p = 0,05

114

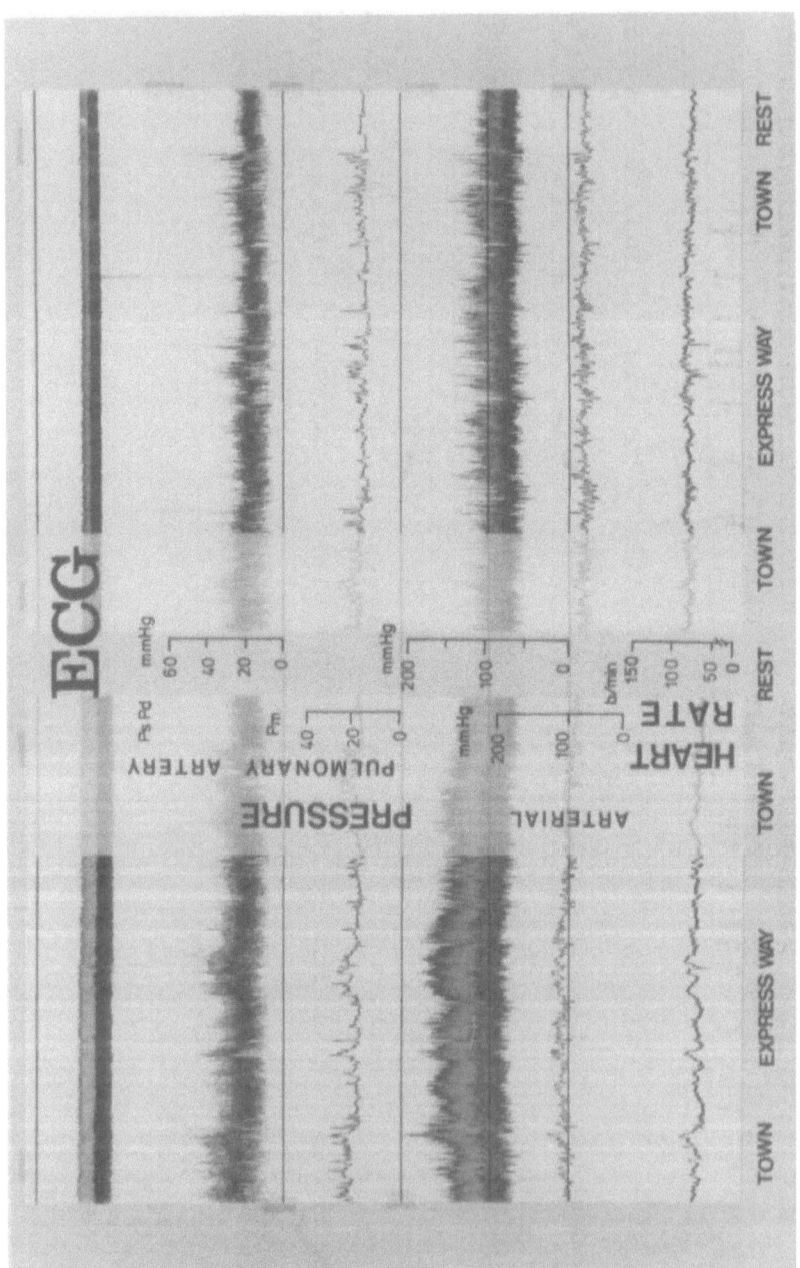

Figure 6. Radiotransmission of the electrocardiogram and continuous blood pressure measurements in the pulmonary artery and the arterial system in a 59-year old patient with coronary heart disease during driving a car before and after s.l. intake of 10 mg of Isosorbiddinitrate.

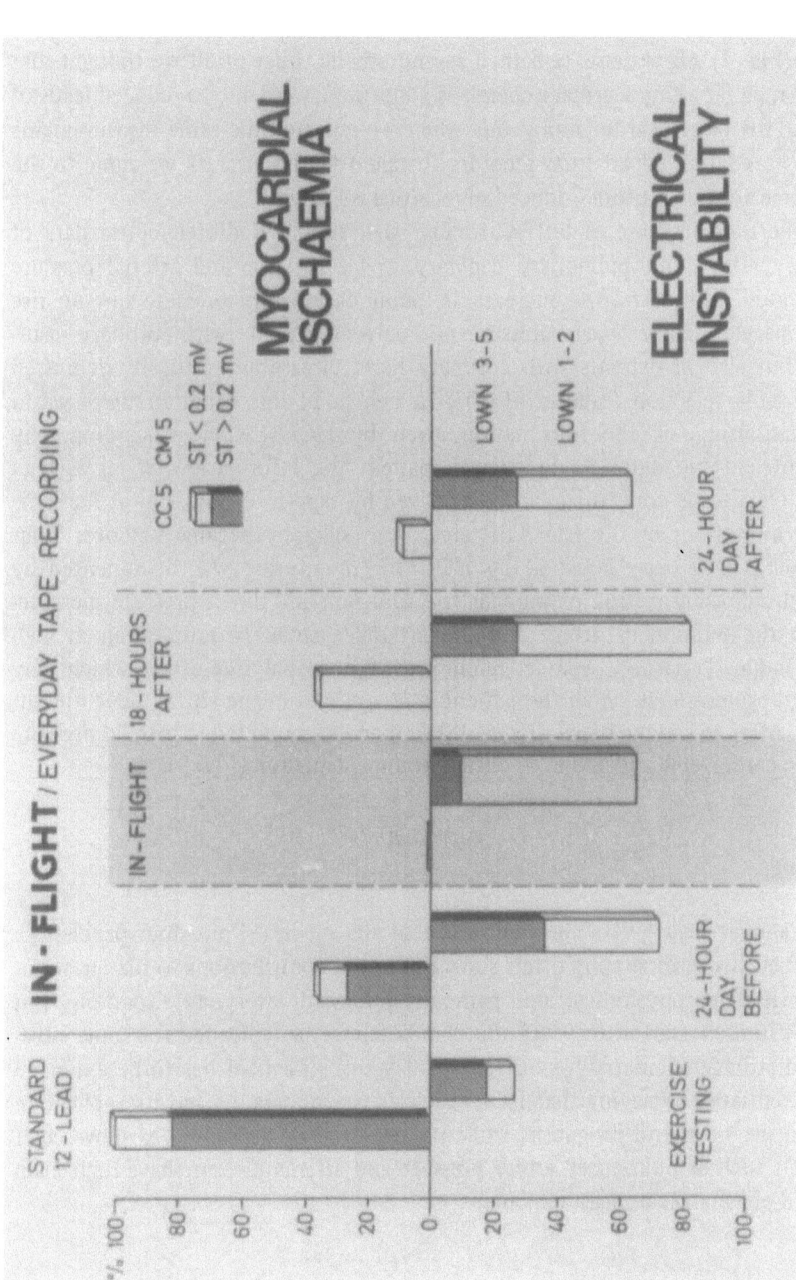

Figure 7. Incidence of ischemic episodes and ventricular ectopic activity in 24 patients with coronary heart disease during bicycle exercise testing, 24-hour HOLTER monitoring during everyday activities and during flights up to 15 000 feet in a non-pressurized aicraft.

ischemia and scar tissue to such a high altitude. Myocardial ischemia, ventricular arrhythmias and left ventricular insufficiency are to be expected due to a drop in arterial saturation from 96.4% at 1011 feet airport elevation to 87.3% at 10 000 feet and 75.3% at 15 000 feet down to 63.4% at 19 000 feet. In comparison with a 24-hour HOLTER electrocardiography the day before and after the flight, the recordings − contrary to expectation − demonstrated in this extreme situation unexpectedly neither myocardial ischemia nor increase in ventricular ectopic activity. (Fig. 7) All patients remained asymptomatic. First of all we thought that these data, as far as myocardial ischemia is concerned, were due to reduced leads of the HOLTER electrocardiography but when we repeated the same measurements with the standard 12-lead ECG-recorder installed in the aircraft we came to the same conclusion: no altitude-induced myocardial ischemia.

Was there no increase of left ventricular wall stress? Radiotelemetric data of pulmonary artery and pulmonary capillary wedge pressure and arterial pressure demonstrated altitude-related increase in pulmonary artery pressure but no rise in pulmonary capillary wedge pressure not only in patients with coronary insufficiency but also in patients with coronary heart disease and critically depressed left ventricular ejection fraction of 30% or below. In this situation there was a close relationship of the information given by HOLTER electrocardiography and radiotelemetric data. So in a given patient the information as far as high altitude tolerance is concerned can be achieved by tape-recording. But at the same time the limitations of the HOLTER electrocardiography became obvious. What never would have been detected by HOLTER monitoring was documented by combined radiotransmission of the electrocardiogram and direct pressure measurements in the pulmonary artery and the arterial system. Nitrates given at high altitude induce hazardous venous pooling as a potential side-effect which may cause cardiogenic shock when the patient is at rest and in the sitting oder upright position. After s.l. intake of 1 − 10 mg ISDN there is a rapid fall in arterial pressure leading to cardiogenic shock due to critical volume depletion (Fig. 8).

Conclusion

These examples may give some impression of the medical "out-door problems". HOLTER electrocardiography offers some important contributions to the questions dealing with the physiology and pathophysiology of everyday situations. But HOLTER himself started in 1963 that "radiotelemetry is needed for some situations and storage-telemetry for others". Today this statement has to be extended and differentiated by saying that HOLTER electrocardiography has its application mainly in diagnosis and prognosis, while radiotransmission of other cardiovascular parameters such as pulmonary artery pressure and arterial pressure have their main interest in physiological measurements.

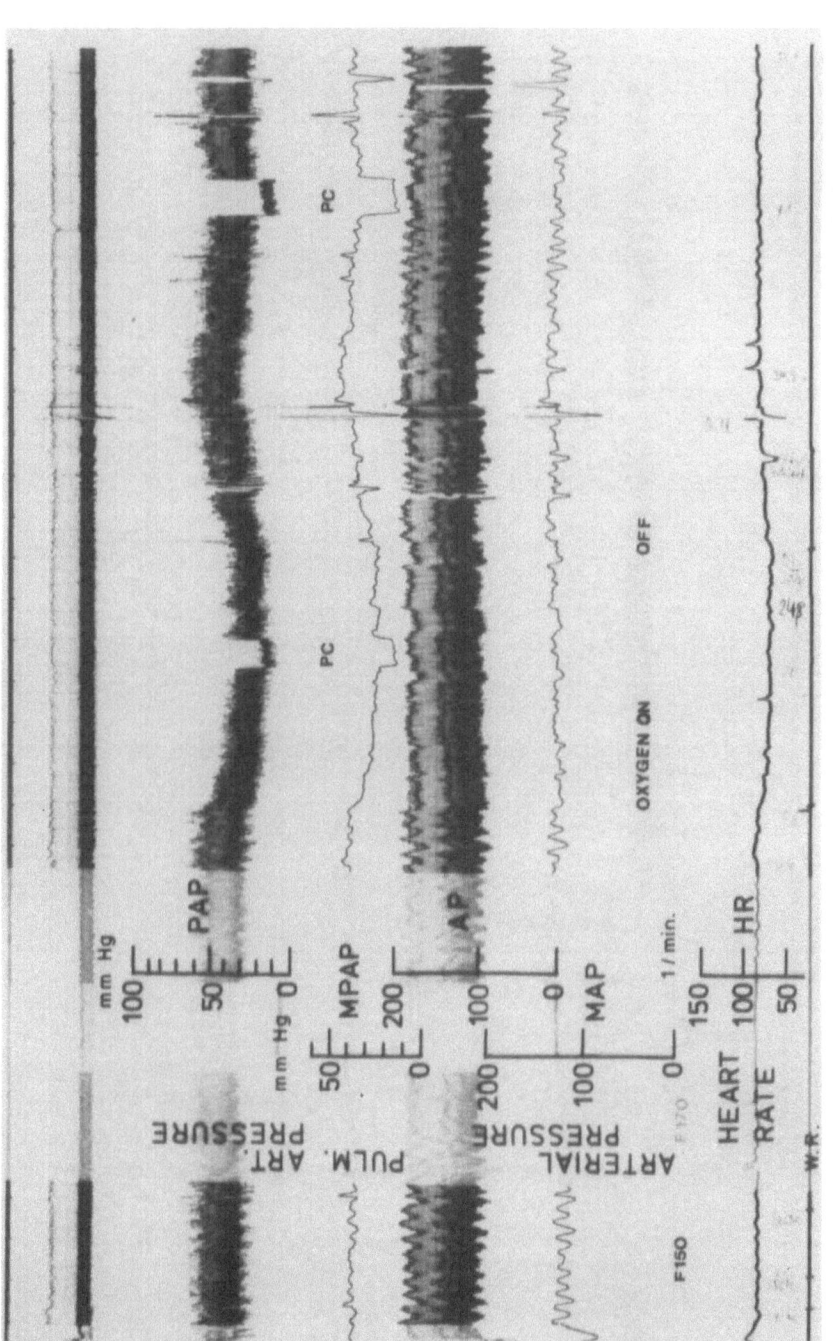

Figure 8. Nitrate-induced cardiogenic shock in a 53-year old coronary patient with aneurysm during air travel at 15 000 feet exposed to actual oxygen pressure in a non-pressurized aicraft.

118

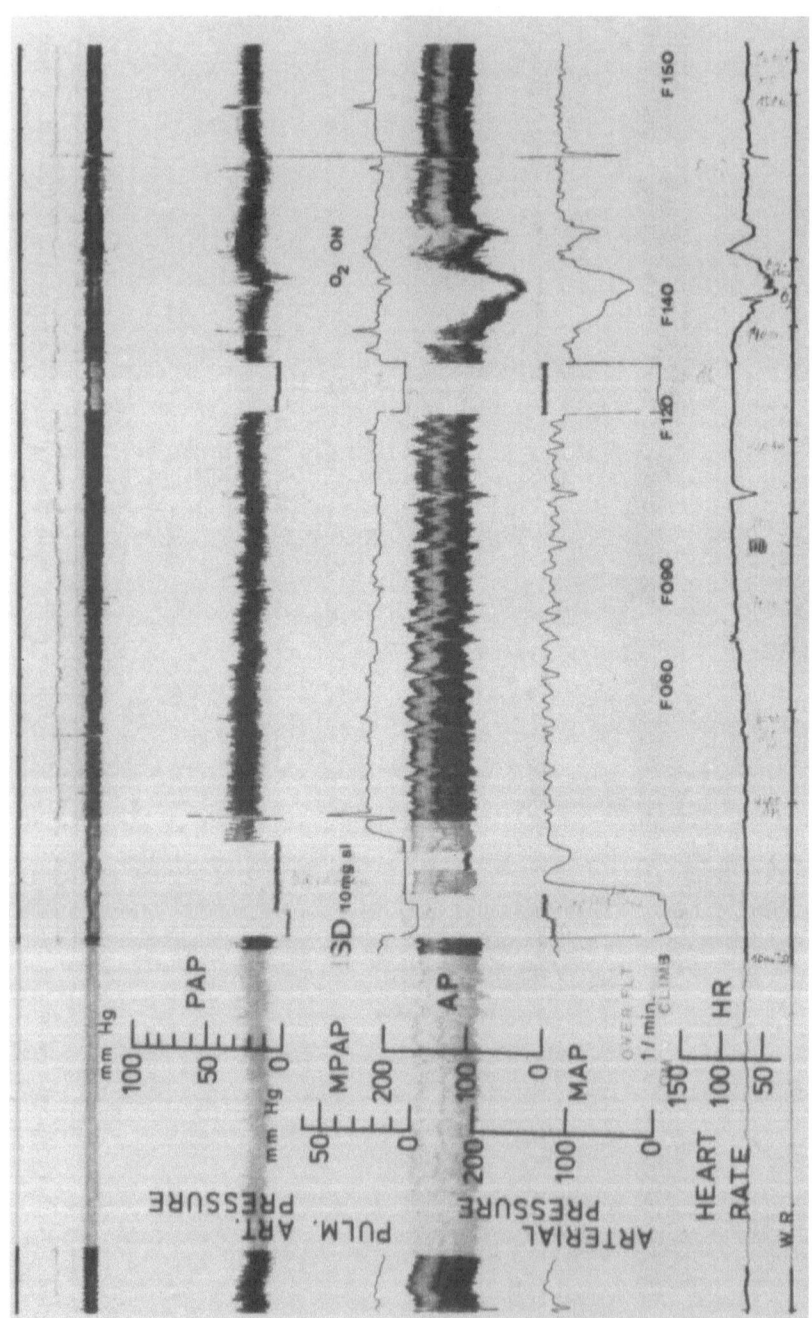

Figure 8b.

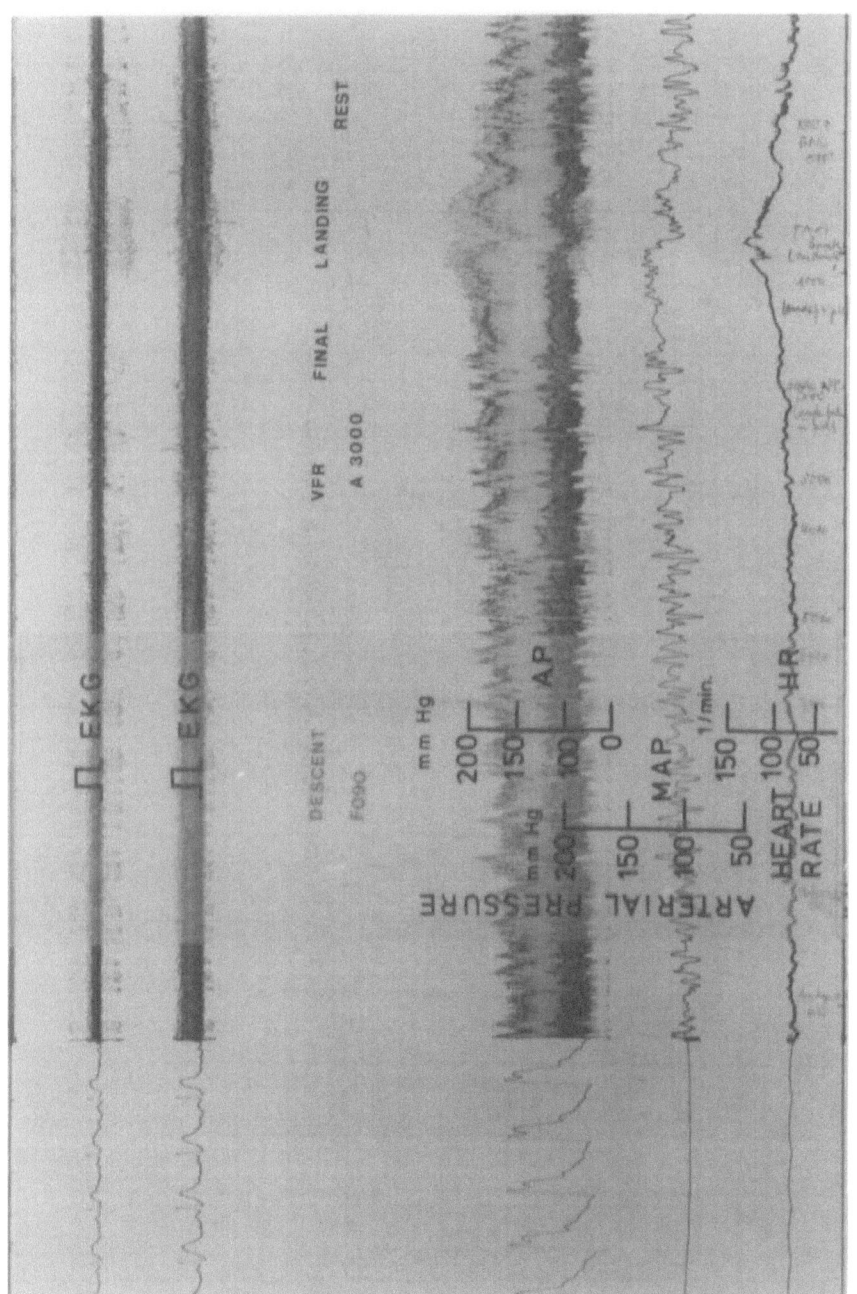

Figure 9a.

120

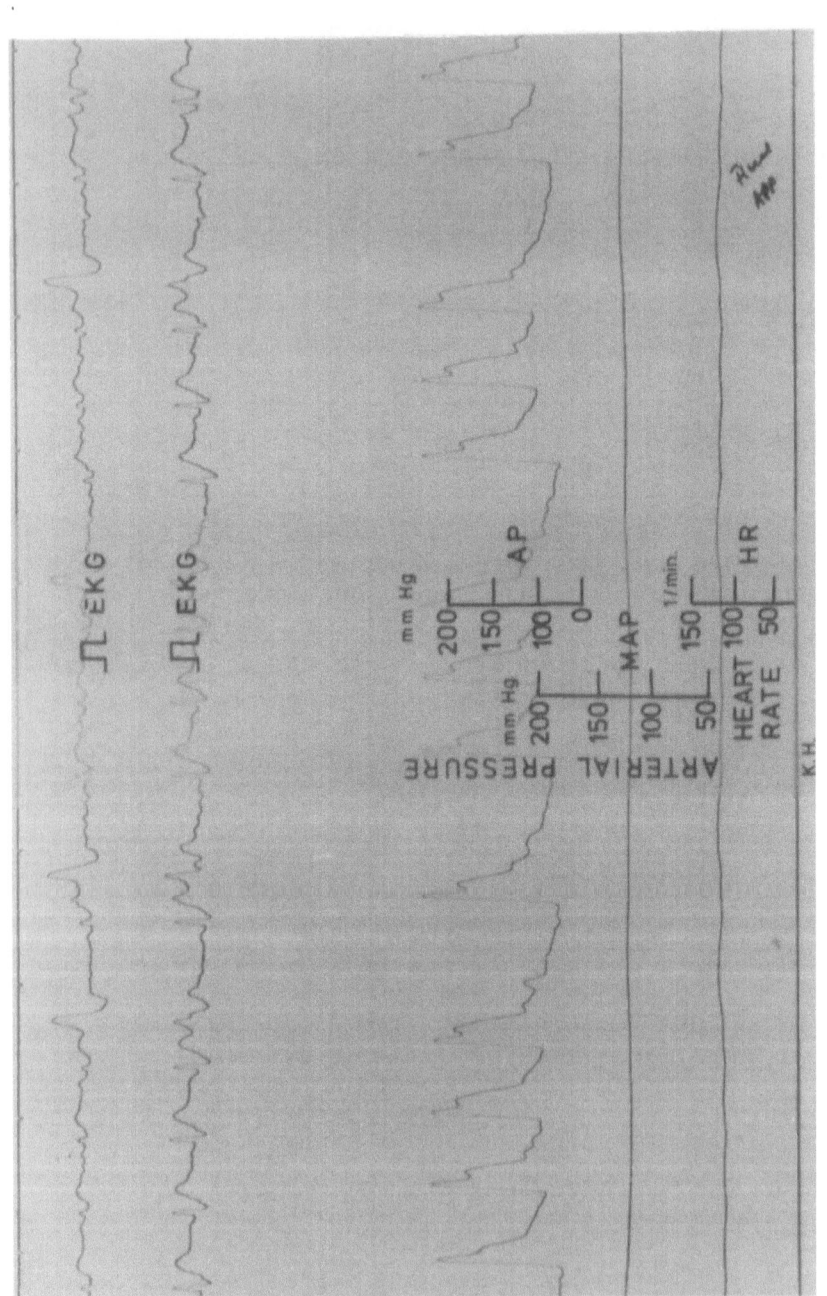

Figure 9b.

Literature

BACHMANN, K. und J. THEBIS
Die drahtlose Übertragung kontinuierlicher direkter Blutdruckmessungen.
Z. Kreislaufforsch. 56, 188 (1967).

BACHMANN, K. und J. THEBIS
Technik und Indikation der arteriellen, pulmonalen und intrakardialen Blutdrucktelemetrie.
4. Jahrestagg. Dtsch. Ges. med. und biol. Elektronik, München 1968.

BACHMANN, K., HOFMANN, H., GÜNTHNER, W., ZERZAWY, R.
Ergebnisse telemetrischer Kreislaufuntersuchungen beim Saunabadevorgang.
Sauna Arch. 9:1 (1971).

BACHMANN, K., ZERZAWY, R., FLEISCHER, H.
Beurteilung von Nitropräparaten bei Koronarkranken im Alltag mittels Telemetrie.
In RUDOLPH, SIEGENTHALER, Nitrate.
Nitratsymp. Stockholm 1975 (Urban und Schwarzenberg, München 1976).

BACHMANN, K., SCHEBELLE, K., ZERZAWY, R., KLEIN, G.
In-flight telemetry in pilots and patients with coronary heart disease.
In KLEWE, KLIMMICH, Biotelemetry IV (Döring, Braunschweig 1978).

BASSEY, E.J. and P.H. FENTEM.
Monitoring physical activity.
In Clinical Ambulatory Monitoring.
Ed. W.A. LITTLER, Chapman and Hall, p. 148, London 1980.

BEVAN, A.T., HONOUR, A.J. and F.H. STOTT.
Direct arterial pressure recording in unrestricted man.
Clin. Sci. 36, 329 (1969).

CORDAY, E., BAZIKA, V., LANG, T.W., PAPPELBAUM, St., GOLD, H. and H. BERNSTEIN.
Detection of phantom arrhythmias and evanescent electrocardiographic abnormalities use of prolonged direct electrocardiocording.
J.A., M.A. 417: 421 (1965).

EINTHOVEN, W.
The télécardiogramme.
Arch. Internat. physiol. 4/132 (1906).

HOLTER, N.J. and J.A. GENGERELLI
Remote recording of physiological data by radio.
Rochy Mtn. Med. Inl. 1949.

HOLTER, N.J.
New method for heart studies.
Science 1214–1220 (1961).

HOLTER, N.J.
Some perspective on telemetry in the biological sciences.
Biotelemetry, Pergamon Press, pp. 61–64.

HOLTER, N.J.
Storage telemetry and sudden death.
In. Biotelemetry eds. H.P. KIMMICH, J.A. VOS, Meander, Leiden 1972, p. 151–167.

LITTLER, W.A., HONOUR, A.J., SLEIGHT, P. and F.D. STOTT.
Continuous recording of direct arterial pressure and electrocardiogram in unrestricted man.
Brit.Med.J., 3, 76 (1972).

LITTLER, W.A.
Continuous ambulatory monitoring of direct arterial pressure.
Clinical Ambulatory Monitoring.
In: ed. LITTLER, W.A., Chapman and Hall, London 1980, p. 96–121.

PREVALENCE OF CARDIAC ARRHYTHMIAS IN THE NORMAL ACTIVE POPULATION

V. MANGER CATS AND D. DURRER

Introduction

The first long term ambulatory electrocardiographic recordings in normal subjects are described in 1964 by Gilson and co-workers from Holters group in a study subtitled: "tentative standards and typical patterns" and mainly concerned with technical details of the recorder and interpretational problems of the recorded signal (1). They report on a group of 65 healthy men and women in age groups 25 to 55+, used a one-channel recorder during five hours and noted ventricular premature beats (VPB) in 4 subjects (6%). No mention is made of multiform or repetitive types of VPB.

The next report is from Hinkle and co-workers in 1969 (2). They studied a random selection of 301 men 53 – 60 years old, who had been fully employed for 27 years by the New Jersey Bell Telephone Company. The presence of disease did not lead to exclusion. Six hour recordings with a one-channel device were made "under standard conditions of position, activity, food intake and sleep" including a Valsalva maneuver, a two-step test and the drinking of 500 cc ice water followed by 500 cc of hot coffee. This is the only study with a follow-up. Because of the relatively non selective nature of recruitment it was possible to study several subgroups which led amongst others to a comparison of the prognostic significance of VPB in subjects with and without coronary heart disease in the original sample (3) and an observation about the prognostic significance of slow heart rates (4).

Since 1975 at least 20 reports have been published about cardiac arrhythmias in normal subjects (5–24). In this chapter the results of these studies will be discussed and compared with our own experience in 300 apparently healthy middle aged men.

Apparently Healthy Middle Aged Men

We studied 300 consecutive participants in the coronary risk factor screening program of a national bank. The subjects filled an angina pectoris questionnaire including daily cigarette consumption and present medication. Length, weight and blood pressure were taken and a standard 12-lead ECG was made. A physical examination was performed by the banks physician.

Exclusion criteria were: 1) angina pectoris according to the questionnaire, 2) history of prior myocardial infarction or signs of old myocardial infarction on the ECG, 3) use of β-blocking, anti-anginal or anti-arrhythmic drugs and 4) otherwise kown heart disease.

A two-channel 24-hour Oxford Medilog recorder was used and tapes were analyzed by a full time technician on a Oxford Medilog-1 analyser. From every type of arrhythmia, including maximal and minimal heart rate, at least one write-out at paper speed 25 mm/second was made for documentation and further analysis. The analyst filled a special protocol form, whether or not she had found the following arrhythmias: atrial premature beats, runs of 3 or more atrial premature beats, AV junctional mechanism, ventricular premature beats (VPB), multiform VPB, VPB in bigeminy and runs of VPB and SA or AV conduction disturbances. Because of the semi-automatic nature of the analysis procedure early cycle VPB were not looked for.

What is Normal?

Absence of cardiac disease at first seems a reasonable prerequisite for normality. But at what cost for the subject should the cardiologist go to prove this absence? Few would advocate coronary arteriography. But even a non invasive procedure like the exercise test introduces its own problems: what is the meaning of a so called positive exercise test in subjects without cardiac complaints; what is the incidence of false positive tests in a given age group without complaints; and precisely which electrocardiographic criterion does one choose for positivity? Secondly, with advancing age more subjects will suffer from (sub)clinical cardiac disease. The prevalence of mild but typical angina pectoris in a group of apparently healthy subjects over 75 is reported as high as 33% (20). Parallel with this increase in mild cardiac symptoms runs an increase in electrocardiographic abnormalities which may reflect a normal aging process rather than increased prevalence of cardiac disease (25). Thirdly, abnormal findings during cardiological screening procedures in symptom-free individuals may have an other (prognostic) meaning than the same abnormal finding in a symptomatic patient, as has been demonstrated by Rose (26).

An illustration of different approaches in defining normality is shown in table 1, where the frequency of the used criteria as stated in 22 studies is listed.

It will be appreciated that for example recruitment from a group of general

Table 1. Criteria for normality (22 studies).

Absence of cardiac complaints	19
Normal standard electrocardiogram	17
Normal physical examination and RR	17
No abnormal cardiovascular signs	12
No systemic disease	12
Normal chest röntgenogram	10
No use of chronic medication	7
Normal blood tests	5
Normal echocardiogram	4
Normal exercise test	3
Normal coronary arteriogram	2

practitioners can not lead to as stringent entrance criteria as recruitment from a hospital population. At the other end of this spectrum is the group of patients, referred to a cardiological department, and there, with help of cineangiography and coronary angiography found to be normal. The former group may include some objects with latent cardiac disease, the latter group is highly selected and thus not representative for the common cardiological patient.

Other Differences in Study Design

Most studies use a two-channel 24-hour Holter tape recorder. Early studies sometimes use one-channel equipment with shorter recording times. This can lead to under-estimation of the "true" incidence of arrhythmias (14, 24, 27, 28) and may influence the prognostic value of some of these findings. Reports from large samples of asymptomatic subjects show that the prevalence of VPB in the standard 12-lead electrocardiogram increases with age (29). During prolonged electrocardiographic recording the same trend has been found (3, 6, 10, 19, 24). Therefore samples should be limited to one age group, because mean values from a group composed of teen-agers and octogenarians will give an outcome that is not "normal" for any of the two.

Also, the most meaningful way to present the data has yet to be found. Some concentrate on the maximal frequency of VPB as found in a certain time period or during a chosen number of normal beats, others use a preset definition of frequent VPB and add multiformity, repetitive patterns and early-cycle VPB. Probably the two methods have to be combined, as advocated by Bigger (30).

Dynamics of Normal Sinus Rhythm

Differences between studies in the way the sinus rate is computed make comparison often difficult. Some use the frequency found in three successive RR-intervals

(9, 22), others use the mean frequency over longer periods (16, 19).

The lowest reported heart rate in infants is 59/– (11). In schoolchildren (23), young adults (9, 22) and in our study of middle aged men the lowest heart rates are between 33/– and 40/–. Djiane (19) finds lowest heart rates of 45–47/– in three different age groups but computes mean heart rate from 10 minutes of registration.

In young men and women 24% and 8% showed heart rates below 40/– (9, 22). In middle aged men we found 4% with heart rates below 40/– and 44% with heart rates below 50/–. Clee (17) found a heart rate below 50/– in only one of 50 subjects over 60 years and Camm (20) reports a heart rate of 50/– or less in 10% of subjects 75 years and older.

Lowest heart rates are always found during sleep and most often during sinus arrhythmia. The relatively high incidence of slow heart rates in young adults probably reflects the ability to produce sinus arrhythmia rather than specifically slow heart rates.

The maximal heart rate reported in infants is 220/– (11), in school children 195/– (23), in young adults 180–189/– (9, 22) and in our study 188/–. We found that 49% of subjects had maximal heart rates above 130/–, while Camm (20) found none above 130/– in subjects over 75 and Djiane (19) reports 126/– as the maximal heart rate in 25 subjects over 65 years old. Camm (20) also noted that 35 tapes revealed sinus rates which did not vary by more than 10 beats per minute throughout the 24 hours. This decreasing variability of the heart rate with increasing age has also been described by Kostis (31).

Although changes in life style probably also influence maximal heart rate the lower maximal heart rates found in older age seem to reflect a diminished capacity of the sinus node to generate faster rates. This, of course, is well known in exercise cardiology.

Pauses in sinus rhythm of more than 2.5 seconds were not found in 826 men and women between the age of 7 and 86 years old (9, 19, 22, 23, 32) including our own study. Djiane (19) describes 66% pauses between 1.5 and 2.5 seconds in 29 subjects under 30 years, 24% pauses in 21 subjects between 30 and 57 years and 4% pauses in 25 subjects over 65. In other studies sinus nodal dysfunction is not discussed. We have found no reports of well established second or third degree sino-atrial block during Holter tape registration in samples of normal subjects. Thus, it seems that pauses less than 2.5 seconds during sinus rhythm also reflect the age linked ability to produce sinus arrhythmia rather than a true arrest of sinus nodal activity.

Supraventricular Ectopic Activity

Isolated atrial premature beats are reported in 19–92% of normal subjects (5, 6, 9, 10, 16, 19, 20, 22, 23). This incidence is not age related.

Runs of 3 or more atrial premature beats are found in 2% of young men (9) and 4% of young women (22). Three studies in age groups 16 to 80 (6, 7, 10) report incidences of 4–9%. Baxter (16) noted single brief episodes of supraventricular tachycardia in 4 of 60 (6.6%) car workers 40 to 59 years old. We found runs of 3 or more atrial premature beats in 20% of middle aged men. Djiane (19) found no subjects with such runs under 30 years of age, one in 21 subjects between 30 and 57 and at least 8 in 25 subjects over 65 years of age.

Most authors agree that runs are seldom longer than 20 beats in a row and runs are mostly slower than 180/–.

Atrial fibrillation or -flutter is not reported in the younger age groups. Verbaan (10) reports an incidence of 3% atrial fibrillation in a group of subjects 20–80 years old. Djiane (19) found atrial fibrillation exclusively in 4 of 25 subjects over 65. Camm (20) found 8 subjects with permanent and 3 with paroxysmal atrial fibrillation in 106 normal subjects over 75 in 9 of whom the standard electrocardiogram had already revealed atrial fibrillation. We found atrial fibrillation and atrial flutter in 4 of 178 subjects 50 to 59 years old and none in the subjects 40 to 49 years old.

From these studies one can conclude that the prevalence of runs of 3 or more atrial premature beats increases with age and that unexpected atrial fibrillation probably only occurs over the age of 50.

AV-junctional mechanism as at least one AV-junctional escape beat was observed in 22% of young men (9). In young women (22) only 2 subjects (4%) had AV-junctional escape beats and one of them showed an episode of six beats of "accelerated" AV-junctional rhythm. Clarke (7) found episodes of AV-junctional rhythm in two successive 24-hour Holter tape recordings in 8 of 86 subjects age 16 to 65. Six of them were under 40. No mention is made of the frequency of the rhythm or the age distribution in the selected group. Glasser (18) describes one subject with "ectopic junctional" rhythm in a group of 13 subjects age 60 to 84 and Camm (20) finds AV-junctional premature beats in 3%, AV-junctional escape beats in 4% and AV-junctional tachycardia in 2% of 106 subjects above 75 years. In this group of older subjects no slow sustained AV-junctional rhythms were observed.

We found repeated episode of 3 or more beats of AV-junctional rhythm with a frequency of 43–104/– in 10 subjects without apparent heart disease. AV-junctional tachycardia was not found in our group of normal subjects.

On the basis of these studies one can conclude that AV-junctional escape beats occur in 22% of young male adults and that a slow AV-junctional rhythm in later life not always indicates serious cardiac disease.

Conduction Disturbances

Sino-atrial block is described by Southall (11) in one infant in the first two weeks of life. It later disappeared. We have not been able to find in the available literature an unmistakable case of second or third degree sino-atrial block later in life in normal subjects during Holter tape registration. As mentioned above, sinus pauses of more than 2.5 seconds were not reported in larger groups of normal subjects.

First degree AV-block was found in 9 of 91 school children (10%) 7 to 11 years old (23). It was noted in 8% of young men (9) and 12% of young women (22). Clarke (7) found one of 86 subjects, a 35 year old man, with first degree AV-block and Clee (17) found it in one of 50 subjects over 60. We found first degree AV-block in 8 of 300 subjects (2.7%).

Second degree AV-block was found in 3% of school children (23), in 4–6% of young adults (9, 22) and in 4% of subjects over 60 (17).

We found episodes of second degree AV-block in 2% of middle aged men.

Third degree AV-block as an unexpected finding was recorded only once in a total number of 722 normal subjects (including our own study) age 7 to 95 years in which AV-block is discussed (7, 9, 17, 18, 19, 20, 22, 23). This case was reported by Camm (20) in his study of active elderly subjects over 75.

Ventricular Premature Beats

In 1964 Gilson, Holter and Glasscock (1) using a one-channel 5-hour tape recorder "noted ventricular ectopic beats, however, in only 4 of 65 (6%) normal subjects". Since then VPB have been the main interest of almost every study with Holter tape recording. While in postmyocardial infarction patients the prognostic value of so called "complex" VPB has been established in several studies, the only published follow-up in normal subjects is Hinkle's study of 301 actively employed american men (2). More follow-up data are clearly needed in normal subjects because the prognostic value of a VPB in a normal subject is not necessarily the same as in a patient who suffered a myocardial infarction.

The term "complex" VPB in this chapter defines any of the following:
1. Frequent VPB (frequent as defined in original publication)
2. Multiform VPB
3. Ventricular couplets
4. Runs of 3 or more VPB

In 80 infants Southall (11) found 78 to be free of VPB; one had isolated VPB and another had "multiple" VPB. However, these 80 infants were selected because of absence of arrhythmias on a standard ECG and served as a control group for 23 infants with arrhythmias on a standard ECG selected from a group of 1212. Six of these 23 had VPB during Holter tape registration. Complex VPB (three times ventricular tachycardia and once VPB in bigeminy) were detected in 4 of these 23 infants with arrhythmias on the standard ECG, but not in 80 infants with normal standard ECG. All ventricular arrhythmias had disappeared at the age of six months.

In school children Southall (23) found 91 of 92 to be free of VPB. One had isolated VPB (less than 1/hour). No complex VPB were found.

The age group 20 to 29 years is studied by several authors. Engel (5) found no VPB in 69% of 35 young men and women with a mean age of 24 ± 4 years during a one-channel recording of about 7.5 hours. Nine subjects had low frequency VPB (less than 12/−). One had frequent VPB (more than 12/−) and one subject had multiform VPB and VPB in couplets. Two subjects (6%) thus had complex VPB.

Bethge (12) studied 24 airforce soldiers with a mean age of 21 during 10 hours of rest and found only low frequency VPB in one and no VPB in the others. The 24 soldiers served as controls for a group of 20 patients who underwent diagnostic left ventricular angiography and coronary arteriography and were found to be normal. Nineteen of the patients showed low frequency (less than 5 VPB/hour) while one had frequent VPB (more than 5 VPB/hour). No complex VPB were found. Brodsky (9) made 24-hour two-channel Holter tape recordings in 50 male medical students age 23 to 27 and found no VPB in 25. From the others 24 had low frequency VPB and one had frequent VPB (more than 50 VPB/24 hours); of them 6 had multiform VPB, one subject had coupled VPB and one subject had an episode of ventricular tachycardia (5 beats) but no VPB in the rest of his recording.

At least 7 and possibly 9 subjects had complex VPB in this group.

Djiane (19) studied 29 subjects below 30 years of age with a one-channel 24-hour Holter tape recording and found low frequency VPB in 5 of them, while 2 of those 5 had coupled VPB. Complex forms were thus found in 2/29 (7%).

Sobotka (22) made 24 hour two-channel recordings in 50 young women age 22 to 28, found no VPB in 23, low frequency VPB in 22, frequent VPB (more than 50/24 hours) in 3, multiform in 5 and ventricular tachycardia (3 beats) in one subject. At least 5 and possibly 9 subjects had complex VPB in this study.

If we pool these studies of 188 subjects 20 to 29 years old, we find that 46−96% has no detectable VPB and 0−14 or 18% has complex forms of VPB.

This age group of 20 to 29 years, the young adults, will now be compared with *the age group of 40 to 59 years*, the middle aged.

Verbaan (10) studied 38 subjects 41 to 60 years old with two-channel 24-hour recording and found no VPB in 21%, only uniform VPB in 39.5% and multi-form, R on T and repetitive forms of VPB in 39.5%.

Federman (13), using one-channel 24-hour recording in a control group of 21 normal subjects found 11 (52%) to be free of VPB, while 4 (19%) had frequent VPB (more than one VPB/10 normal beats). No multiform or repetitive VPB were detected. Poblete (15) found no VPB in 67% of 30 middle aged asymptomatic volunteers, infrequent VPB (less then 10/30 minutes) in 5 (17%) and complex forms in another 4 (13%).

Baxter (16) made 24-hour recordings in 60 car workers age 40 to 59 and found no VPB in 65%, multiform VPB in 10% and coupled VPB in 6.6%.

If we pool these studies of 149 middle aged subjects we find that 21−65% has no detectable VPB and 10−39.5% has complex forms. This suggests, with advancing age, a decrease in the number of subjects without VPB and an increase in the number of subjects with complex forms of VPB.

Individual studies concerned with wider age ranges confirm this trend (3, 6, 10,

Table 2. Ventricular premature beats in 300 normal men age 40–59: all classes.

0	No VPB	68	(22.7%)
1	VPB < 10/30 minutes	187	(62.3%)
2	VPB ⩾ 10/30 minutes	43	(14.3%)
3	Multiform VPB	102	(34.0%)
4	VPB in couplets	40	(13.3%)
5	VPB in runs ⩾ 3	5	(1.7%)

Table 3. Ventricular premature beats in 300 normal men age 40–59: maximal class only.

0	No VPB	68	(22.7%)
1	VPB < 10/30 minutes	116	(38.7%)
2	VPB ⩾ 10/30 minutes	8	(2.7%)
3	Multiform VPB	65	(21.7%)
4	VPB in couplets	38	(12.7%)
5	VPB in runs ⩾ 3	5	(1.7%)

19, 24).

Our findings in 300 apparently healthy middle aged men are shown in tables 2 and 3.

We found no detectable VPB in 68 (22.7%) and complex forms in at least 116 (38.7%). These results closely resemble the findings of Verbaan (10) in the same age group. One explanation for the close resemblance of our findings and the difference with other studies may be that we use the same type of equipment, analyse according to the same protocol and work in the same (small) country.

Why we find more complex forms than most other studies is not clear, but does not necessarily follow from our selection procedure, for we were also able to detect more complex VPB in postmyocardial infarction patients than are usually reported (33).

It is clear, however, that more studies have to be executed in larger samples of normal subjects, limited to one age group, to establish reliable "normal values" for the Holter tape laboratory. On the basis of our experience with normal subjects and postmyocardial infarction patients, we think that even some complex forms of VPB may be normal in middle age.

It may be that the underlying pathology has more prognostic value than ventricular premature beats found during Holter tape registration. Or, as it has been said by Goldstein (34): "It may be . . . that the ventricular premature beat is like the bullet in a game of biological 'russian roulette' . . . if it occurs in a metabolic setting or clinical state which can lead to electrical dysorganization".

Acknowledgement

The study of 300 apparently healthy middle aged men was supported by grant nr. 77.083 from the Dutch Heart Foundation.

We wish to thank Hélène Heyen for her expert help in analyzing the tape recordings and Pia Botman for preparing the manuscript.

References

1. Gilson JS, Holter NJ, Glasscock WR. Clinical observations during the Electrocardiocorder-AVSEP continuous Electrocardiographic system. Am J Cardiol 14: 204–217, 1964.
2. Hinkle LE, Carver ST, Stevens M. The frequency of asymptomatic disturbances of cardiac rhythm and conduction in middle-aged men. Am J Cardiol 24: 629–650, 1969.
3. Hinkle LE, Carver ST, Argyros DC. The prognostic significance of ventricular premature contractions in healthy people and people with coronary heart disease. Acta Cardiologica (Suppl.) 18: 5–32, 1974.
4. Hinkle LE, Carver ST, Plakun A. Slow heart rate and increased risk of cardiac death in middle aged men. Arch Intern. Med 129: 732–748, 1972.
5. Engel UR, Burckhardt D. Häufigkeit und Art von Herzrhythmusstörungen sowie EKG-veränderungen bei jugendlichen herzgesunde Probanden. Schweiz Med Wschr 105: 1467–1469, 1975.
6. Raftery EB, Cashman PMM. Long-term recording of the electrocardiogram in a normal population. Postgrad Med J 52 (Suppl. 7): 32–37, 1976.
7. Clarke JM, Shelton JR, Hamer J, Taylor S, Venning GR. The rhythm of the normal human heart. Lancet II: 508–512, 1976.
8. Kennedy HL, Underhill SJ. Frequent or complex ventricular ectopy in apparently healthy subjects. Am J Cardiol 38: 141–148, 1976.
9. Brodsky M, Wu D, Denes P, Kanakis C, Rosen KM. Arrhythmias documented by 24 hour continuous electrocardiographic monitoring in 50 male medical students without apparent heart disease. Am J Cardiol 39: 390–395, 1977.
10. Verbaan CJ, Pool J, van Wanrooij J. Incidence of cardiac arrhythmias in a presumed healthy population in: Proceedings of the second international symposium on ambulatory monitoring (Scott FD, Sleight P, Raftery EB, Goulding L, Eds). Academic Press, London p: 1–5, 1978.
11. Southall DP, Orrell MJ, Talbot JF, Brinton RJ, Vulliamy DG, Johnson AM, Keeton BR, Anderson RH, Shinebourne EA. Study of cardiac arrhythmias and other forms of conduction abnormality in new born infants. Brit Med J 2: 597–599, 1977.
12. Bethge KP, Bethge HC, Graf A, van den Berg E, Lichtlen P. Kammer-Arrhythmien bei chronisch koronarer Herzkrankheit. Z Kardiol 66: 1–9, 1977.
13. Federman J, Whitford JA, Anderson ST, Pitt A. Incidence of ventricular arrhythmias in first year after myocardial infarction. Brit Heart J 40: 1243–1250, 1978.
14. Kennedy HL, Chandra V, Saythers KL, Caralis DG. Effectiveness of increasing hours of continuous ambulatory electrocardiography in detecting maximal ventricular ectopy. Am J Cardiol 42: 925–930, 1978.
15. Poblete PF, Kennedy HL, Caralis DG. Detection of ventricular ectopy in patients with coronary heart disease and normal subjects by exercise testing and ambulatory electrocardiography. Chest 74: 402–407, 1978.
16. Baxter PJ, White WG, Barnes GM, Cashman PMM. Ambulatory electrocardiography in car workers. Brit J Ind Med 35: 99–103, 1978.

132

17. Clee MD, Smith N, McNeill GP, Wright DS. Dysrhythmias in apparently healthy elderly subjects. Age and Ageing 8: 173–176, 1979.
18. Glasser SP, Clark PI, Applebaum HJ. Occurrence of frequent complex arrhythmias detected by ambulatory monitoring. Chest 75: 565–568, 1979.
19. Djiane P, Egré A, Bory M, Savin B, Mostefa S, Serradimigni A. L'enregistrement électrocardiographique chez les sujets normaux. Arch Mal Coeur 72: 655–661, 1979.
20. Camm AJ, Evans KE, Ward DE, Martin A. The rhythm of the heart in active elderly subjects. Am Heart J 99: 598–603, 1980.
21. Hogstedt C, Söderholm B, Bodin L. 48-Hour ambulatory electrocardiography in dynamite workers and controls. Brit J Ind Med 37: 299–306, 1980.
22. Sobotka PA, Mayer JH, Bauernfeind RA, Kanakis C, Rosen KM. Arrhythmias documented by 24-hour continuous ambulatory electrocardiographic monitoring in young women without apparent heart disease Am Heart J 101: 753–759, 1981.
23. Southall DP, Johnston F, Shinebourne EA, Johnston PGB. 24-Hour electrocardiographic study of heart rate and rhythm patterns in population of healthy children. Brit Heart J 45: 281–291, 1981.
24. Kostis JB, McCrone K, Moreyra AE, Gotzoyannis S, Aglitz NM, Natarajan N, Kuo PT. Premature ventricular complexes in the absence of identifiable heart disease. Circulation 63: 1351–1356, 1981.
25. Fisch C. Electrocardiogram in the Aged: An independent marker of heart disease? Am J Medicine 70: 4–6, 1981.
26. Rose G, Baxter PJ, Reid DD, McCartney P. Prevalence and prognosis of electrocardiographic findings in middle-aged men. Brit Heart J 40: 636–643, 1978.
27. Lown B, Wolf M. Approaches to sudden death from coronary heart disease. Circulation 44: 130–42, 1971.
28. Winkle RA, Peters F, Hall R. Characterization of ventricular tachyarrhythmias on ambulatory ECG recordings in post-myocardial infarction patients: arrhythmia detection and duration of recording, relationship between arrhythmia frequency and complexity and day-to-day reproducability. Am Heart J 102: 162–169, 1981.
29. Hiss RG, Averill KH, Lamb LE. Electrocardiographic findings in 67, 375 asymptomatic subjects. III ventricular rhythms. Am J Cardiol 6: 96–107, 1960.
30. Bigger JT, Weld FM. Analysis of prognostic significance of ventricular arrhythmias after myocardial infarction. Brit Heart J 45: 717–724, 1981.
31. Kostis JB, Aglitz N, Amendo MT, DiPietro J, Moreyra AE, Kuo PT. The diurnal variation of heart rate in normal subjects; effects of age. Chest (Abstr.) 76: 357, 1979.
32. Bjerregaard P. The longest pauses observed during ambulatory electrocardiography in healthy subjects. VIII European Congress of Cardiology (Abstr.): 83, Karger, 1980.
33. Manger Cats, V, Lie KI, van Capelle FJL, Durrer D. Limitations of 24 hour ambulatory electrocardiographic recording in predicting coronary events after acute myocardial infarction. Am J Cardiol 44: 1257–1262, 1979.
34. Goldstein S. Sudden death and coronary heart disease. Futura Publishing Company, Inc. Mt. Kisco, New York, page 81, 1974.

THE SPONTANEOUS VARIABILITY OF VENTRICULAR ARRHYTHMIAS

STUART J. CONNOLLY, ROGER A. WINKLE

Introduction

During the past decade there has been a great increase in the use of prolonged ambulatory ECG monitoring for the determination of antiarrhythmic drug efficacy and for the prediction of prognosis in patients with ischemic heart disease. As with any diagnostic procedure, reproducibility of the test in the same patient is highly desirable. There is now ample evidence that considerable variation of ventricular arrhythmias may occur from minute-to-minute and day-to-day. The lack of complete reproducibility of ambulatory monitoring is in large part due to the inherent biological variability which chronic ventricular arrhythmias manifest. Therefore refinement of the technology to give more accurate tape analysis cannot be expected to improve the reproducibility of this test. The lack of reproducibility of ambulatory monitoring limits the usefulness of this test. However, by understanding the limitations of a test one can interpret the results properly and avoid overinterpretation. In this chapter we shall examine the phenomenon of spontaneous variability of ventricular arrhythmias and assess the impact this has on the use of ambulatory monitoring to assess drug efficacy and to predict prognosis. We shall also take a brief look at some factors which may cause this variability.

Variation in VPB Frequency

In the first article to comment specifically on VPB variation Myburgh and Van Gelder concluded that there was a considerable degree of constancy over time in VPB frequency in their patients (1). This study was not specifically designed to examine the problem of variability, and indeed there was considerable variation in some patients. For example, 16 of 19 patients who had no VPB's on the initial 6 hour recording had VPB's on a subsequent recording 6 to 42 months later. In contrast to this report most other reports have concluded that marked variation in ventricular arrhythmias does occur over time.

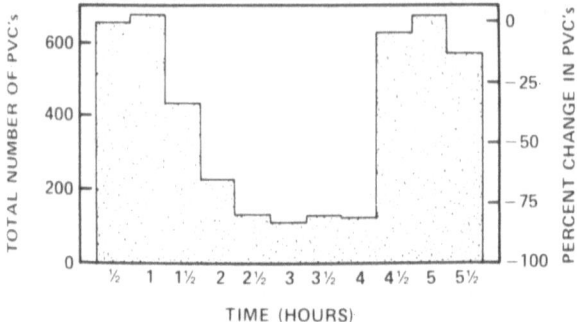

Figure 1. A patient with marked spontaneous half-hour to half-hour variation (from Winkle RA. 1978. Circulation 57: 1116–1121).

An early report concerning VPB variability analyzed the half-hour to half-hour variability in the frequency of VPB's during a five and one-hour hour ambulatory ECG (2). Twenty patients with frequent VPB's were studied. The initial half-hour was used as a control period to which subsequent half-hour periods were compared. For the group as a whole there were no significant changes in VPB frequency. For individuals there was great variability in the VPB frequency from half-hour to half-hour. The maximum change seen compared to control in any half-hour was −99% to +1100%. Twelve of 20 patients experienced a 60% reduction in VPB's and 7 experienced an 80% reduction in VPB's in at least one half-hour period. Figure 1 demonstrates the spontaneous variability seen in one patient.

Several studies have investigated whether longer periods of monitoring could reduce the variability seen from hour to hour. Kennedy and co-workers reported 90 patients who had 2 consecutive 24-hour ambulatory ECG's (3). Sixty-seven patients had coronary artery disease and 23 were normal. The authors' approach was to determine if an increase in the rate of detection of very frequent VPB's could be achieved by increasing the monitoring time from 6 hours to 48 hours. Eighty-five percent with very frequent VPB's (60 VPB's/hr) were detected within 24 hours of monitoring and 100% were detected by 36 hours. This type of study underestimates the degree of variation which occurs because it ignores variation occurring from period to period as long as the arrhythmia occurs in the first period. The absence of arrhythmias may be an important finding and the reproducibility of a negative result is equally important as that of a positive result.

Day-to-day VPB variability was assessed in 17 patients participating in an antiarrhythmic drug trial who had two control 24-hour ambulatory ECG's 5 weeks apart (4). All of these patients had frequent VPB's. Nine had ischemic heart disease, 1 mitral valve prolapse and 7 were normal except for their arrhythmias. For the group considered as a whole no significant change occurred. However, individual patients showed marked variation from one 24-hour period to another. In individual patients changes as great as −91% to +198% occurred. Five of the 16 patients analyzed had a spontaneous decline of greater than 50% and one patient was found to have a decline of VPB's of more than 90%.

Pratt and co-workers performed 3 consecutive 24-hour ECG's on 14 patients with stable ischemic heart disease (5). All the patients had frequent VPB's. For the group as a whole the greatest change between any 2 days was 30%. Individual patients showed fluctuations as great as +316% and −79% from one 24-hour period to the next.

Quantitation of VPB Variation

Once the spontaneous variability of ventricular arrhythmias was appreciated, the use of ambulatory ECG to assess antiarrhythmic drug efficacy became problematic. Although wide variations in the frequency of VPB's do occur there is a limit to this variation. Several authors have applied statistical methods to the analysis of prolonged ambulatory monitoring to quantify the degree of variation which occurs. The goal of these studies has been to formulate quidelines for clinical trials of antiarrhythmic drugs in individual patients both with respect to the duration of monitoring needed and the degree of change in arrhythmia frequency required to be confident that the change seen is due to the drug and is not spontaneous.

Morganroth and co-workers were the first to apply an analysis of variance to data acquired from ambulatory monitoring (6). Fifteen patients with frequent VPB's ($\geqslant$ 30/hr over 24 hrs in their 1st 24-hour recording) had three 24-hour ambulatory ECG's. Five patients in this group had a repeat 72-hour recording three months later. They determined the percent reduction in VPB frequency required during a test period to demonstrate a statistically significant ($p \geqslant 0.05$) reduction compared to a control period. As seen in Table 1 if two 8-hour recordings were compared, a 90.3% reduction was required to be 95% confident that the change which occurred was not related to spontaneous variability. If two 24-hour recordings were used an 83.4% reduction was required. If two 72-hour recordings were used a 64.6% reduction was required. An interesting observation was that patients with very frequent VPB's ($>1,000$/hr) manifested a much lower degree of natural variation in the frequency of their VPB's from day to day.

Table 1. Minimal percentage reduction in mean hourly VPB frequency required to demonstrate (with 95% confidence) an effect not attributable to spontaneous variation (from Morganroth J, et al. 1978. Circulation 58: 408–414).

Length of Monitoring	Number of Control	Days Test	Minimal Percent VPB Reduction
8 hours	1	1	−90.3
24 hours	1	1	−83.4
24 hours	3	3	−64.6
24 hours	7	7	−49.3
24 hours	14	14	−38.2

Engler and co-workers arrived at a similar result when they analyzed two consecutive 24-hour control ambulatory ECG's in 18 patients undergoing a drug withdrawal trial. The 95% confidence limit for variation in VPB frequency was a 78% reduction from one day to the next (7).

Sami and co-workers performed an analysis on two 24-hour ambulatory ECG's of 21 patients which were done 2 weeks apart (8). Linear regression analysis was used to determine 95% and 99% confidence limits for variation between the two tapes. A sensitivity threshold (i.e. the minimal frequency of VPB's a patient must have in order for a significant reduction in VPB's to be possible) was also calculated. At low levels of VPB frequency (below the sensitivity threshold) even 100% reduction in VPB's is still within the 95% confidence limits for VPB variability. The percent reduction in VPB frequency necessary to exclude natural variation with 95% confidence decreased as the baseline VPB frequency increased. For patients with frequent VPB's ($\geqslant 30$/hr) a 65% reduction was found to indicate a significant change ($p \leqslant 0.05$). The sensitivity threshold was 2.2 VPB's/hr.

Although there are some differences between these authors with regard to the percent reduction required to exclude spontaneous variation (65% vs. 83%), they all confirm that large reductions in VPB frequency must occur before a change can be attributed to a drug. These studies indicate that there is a trend towards less variability at higher rates of VPB's. Even if prolonged periods of monitoring are used (72 hours), a reduction in VPB's of up to 65% could occur spontaneously.

Complex Ventricular Arrhythmias

Ventricular arrhythmias have been classified in terms of their complexity. Frequent VPB's multifocal VPB's, paired VPB's, ventricular tachycardia, and R on T phenomena are generally considered to be more serious forms of ventricular arrhythmias and have been shown in certain situations to indicate a worse prognosis than infrequent simple VPB's (9). The complexity of VPB's has been shown to exhibit considerable spontaneous variability. In the study of half-hour to half-hour variability during a 5½ hour monitoring period, 15 patients had paired ectopic beats in at least one of the 11 periods. However, only 3 of 15 patients had pairs in each of the 11 periods. Six of 15 patients had pairs in less than half the periods (2).

In another study, two 24-hour ambulatory ECG's done 5 weeks apart were compared in 17 patients (4). The total number of patients exhibiting pairs, bigeminy and ventricular tachycardia was similar for the two recordings. Often, however, individual patients demonstrated a given type of complex VPB in only one recording. As can be seen in Table 2 none of the 5 patients who experienced ventricular tachycardia had it during both 24-hour monitoring periods. Only 5 of 11 patients who were found to have paired VPB's had them on both tapes. This high degree of day-to-day variability is confirmed by the report of Pratt and co-workers (5). In 14 patients who had three consecutive 24-hour ambulatory

Table 2. Reproducibility of each type of complex ventricular arrhythmia on two 24-hour ambulatory ECG's done 5 weeks apart (from Winkle RA, et al. 1978. American Journal of Cardiology 42: 473–480).

	Number of Patients With Arrhythmias		
Type of Arrhythmia	*Both Tests*	*Only One Test*	*Total*
Multifocal	7	4	11
Paired VPB's	5	6	11
Bigeminy	11	4	15
Ventricular tachycardia	0	5	5

ECG's, half the patients who had either paired VPB's or ventricular tachycardia did not have them on at least one 24-hour tape.

Kennedy and co-workers in their study to assess the impact of increasing the duration of monitoring found 21 patients with either paired VPB's, ventricular tachycardia or R on T phenomenon (3). Five of these 21 patients had their complex arrhythmia detected first on the second tape. The authors do not tell us how many had these arrhythmias only on the first tape.

Michaelson and Morganroth used an analysis of variance to quantitate the spontaneous variability of complex ventricular arrhythmias occurring in 20 patients who underwent four 24-hour ambulatory ECG periods (10). All the patients had paired VPB's and 14 had ventricular tachycardia. Confidence limits were derived for variability. If two 24-hour periods are compared a 75% reduction in pairs and a 65% reduction in ventricular tachycardia episodes is required if spontaneous variability is to be excluded with 95% confidence.

Thus it appears that complex grades of ventricular arrhythmias manifest considerable variation from hour-to-hour and from day-to-day. The degree of variation that occurs does not appear to be substantially different from that which affects VPB frequency.

The use of statistical methods has added a degree of sophistication to ambulatory ECG monitoring for measurement of drug effect. However, some of the potentially most important arrhythmias occur infrequently in 24 hours. The use of quantitative methods in this situation is less helpful. For example many patients have paired VPB's or ventricular tachycardia only once or twice a day. In these patients a 65% change is less meaningful. The expense of ambulatory ECG monitoring is high and it tends to make the use of this test more of a research technique, especially for assessing drug efficacy when several 24-hour ambulatory ECG's may be required.

It is important to realize that drug effect is not synonymous with drug efficacy. In other words, although one can detect when a drug causes true changes in the grade and complexity of VPB's, the presence of such changes do not necessarily mean that this drug will prevent sudden death (the ultimate goal of antiarrhythmic therapy directed at PVC suppression).

Table 3. Day-to-day reproducibility of various average hourly VPB frequencies on three consecutive 24-hour ambulatory ECG's in post-myocardial infarction patients (from Winkle RA. et al. American Heart Journal 102: 162–169, 1981).

Average hourly VPB frequency	Number of days				All 3 days the same (3/3 + 0/3)
	3/3	2/3	1/3	0/3	
⩾ 0.5	18	11	8	20	38 (67%)
⩾ 1.0	12	8	11	26	38 (67%)
⩾ 2.0	10	7	7	33	43 (75%)
⩾ 3.0	10	6	3	38	48 (84%)
⩾ 5.0	10	2	4	41	51 (89%)
⩾ 10.0	8	3	3	43	52 (91%)
⩾ 15.0	6	5	3	43	49 (86%)
⩾ 20.0	5	2	5	45	50 (88%)

Numbers in the table refer to number of patients and figures in parentheses refer to percent of the 57 patients.

Post-myocardial Infarction

Ambulatory ECG monitoring in patients after a myocardial infarction is an important tool in predicting prognosis. The presence of complex and frequent ventricular arrhythmias is an indicator of a poor outcome in these patients (9). Several studies have recently assessed the degree of spontaneous variation that occurs in this subset of patients with ventricular arrhythmias, and attempted to determine the optimal monitoring period for the assessment of risk.

Thanavaro and co-workers analyzed 175 single 24-hour ambulatory ECG's in patients who had experienced a myocardial infarction (11). The tapes were recorded prior to hospital discharge and at 2 to 3 months following discharge. The occurrence of complex and of frequent (>30/hr) VPB's in the first and second 12-hour periods were compared. In only 2% of cases did frequent VPB's occur for the first time in the second period. In only 16% and 24% of tapes respectively were paired VPB's and ventricular tachycardia first seen in the second 12-hour period. Although the first 12-hour period appears to detect a large percentage of the important arrhythmias that were discovered, one must realize that the second half-day of recording was uniformly done during sleep, a time when VPB's often undergo a decrease in frequency.

Another study analyzed 3 consecutive 24-hour ECG's from 57 ambulatory patients done between 8 and 11 days following a myocardial infarction (12). Day-to-day reproducibility of VPB frequency was examined. For each patient the number of 24-hour recordings above and below each of the following average hourly VPB frequencies were determined: 0.5, 1.0, 2.0, 3.0, 5.0, 10.0, 15.0 and 20 VPB's per hour. The data (Table 3) suggest that infrequent VPB's are less reproducible than frequent VPB's, since there was perfect day-to-day reproducibility in only 67% of patients for a cutoff VPB frequency of less than 1.0 per hour and 86% to 90% reproducibility for VPB frequencies above 5.0 per hour. However, this apparent increasing reproducibility was in part due to the fact that there were fewer patients with frequent VPB's, and thus the number of patients with all 3 days below a given average VPB frequency (i.e. 0/3) represent a larger proportion of the total. Only 5 of 12 patients who had an average VPB frequency of over 20 on any tape had them on all 3 tapes.

A similar result was found for VPB complexity (Table 4). There was total agreement (presence or absence on all three tapes) in from 63% to 81% of patients for the different types of complex arrhythmias. This was, however, as in the case of VPB frequency, due to the large number of patients free of any specific type of complex arrhythmia. This was most apparent for ventricular tachycardia. Although 81% of patients were correctly classified for the presence or absence of ventricular tachycardia on all three days, among the 12 patients with ventricular tachycardia on at least one tape, 9 had it on only one tape and only one had it on all 3 days.

It would appear that the majority of post-MI patients will be correctly classified as having frequent or infrequent VPB's and as having any given type of complex VPB present or absent from a single 24-hour recording. This correct classification is in large part due to the large number of patients who have infrequent VPB's on all tapes and are free of any given type of VPB on all 3 days. Among the smaller subgroup of patients with frequent VPB's and with each type of complex ventricular arrhythmia, day-to-day variability is greater and a single 24-hour recording may fail to detect many of them.

Table 4. Day-to-day reproducibility of each type of complex VPB on three consecutive 24 hour ambulatory ECG's in post-myocardial infarction patients (from Winkle RA, et al. American Heart Journal 102: 162–169, 1981).

Type of VPB	Number of days				All 3 days the same (3/3 + 0/3)
	3/3	2/3	1/3	0/3	
Multiform	16	9	12	20	36 (63%)
R-on-T	9	6	15	27	36 (63%)
Pairs	4	8	7	38	42 (74%)
Bigeminy	7	5	7	38	45 (79%)
VT	1	2	9	45	46 (81%)
Any complex VPB	24	11	9	12	36 (63%)

Numbers in the table refer to number of patients and figures in parentheses refer to percent of the 57 patients.

Exercise-induced Arrhythmias

Exercise testing has been used to induce ventricular arrhythmias in predisposed subjects. Numerous studies have examined the reproducibility of exercise-induced ventricular arrhythmias. In 1965 Astrand reported on 204 well subjects who had graded exercise tests 8 years apart (13). Of the 7 subjects who had VPB's on exercise, none had them on both tests. In another study 13 patients with frequent VPB's were exercised twice 5 weeks apart (4). The total number of VPB's changed from −100% to +115%. Three of 13 patients (23%) had greater than 90% reduction in VPB's from the first to the second test. There was also a poor reproducibility of VPB complexity between the two tests. For example 9 patients had multifocal VPB's in the first test and only 2 in the second test.

Jelinek and Lown analyzed the multiple exercise tests of 27 post-myocardial infarction patients in a rehabilitation program (14). Over 6 months there was no change in exercise induced arrhythmias for the group as a whole. For individual patients reproducibility was low. Frequent VPB's were reproduced in only 30% of subsequent bicycle tests. Ventricular tachycardia was produced in 50% of subsequent tests.

Faris and co-workers reported their experience with two exercise tests in 543 male policemen performed at an average interval of 2.9 years (15). Eighty-one of the subjects had suspected or definite heart disease. For the whole group ventricular arrhythmias were reproducible; however, individual patients manifested marked variability. In normal subjects there was only a 50% chance of having ventricular arrhythmia on a second test if it was present on the first. In older patients with cardiovascular disease (35 to 54 years) reproducibility of ventricular arrhythmias on the second test was somewhat higher (75%). This difference in reproducibility was statistically significant ($p < 0.05$). There was almost no reproducibility of complex arrhythmias in any group of patients. DeBaker and co-workers also analyzed the exercise-induced arrhythmia reproducibility in normals and found that reproducibility of arrhythmias for the group was high, but for individuals was poor (16).

Shops and co-workers performed 2 exercise tests in 13 patients with exercise-induced ventricular arrhythmias within 45 minutes (17). For the group as a whole there was a reduction in the number of VPB's which could not be explained. In spite of this trend towards a reduction in arrhythmias on the second test, individual patients manifested substantial variability from test to test. Of the 13 patients who had VPB's on the first test, 2 had no VPB's on the second test and 2 others had a greater than 80% reduction on the second test.

Sami and co-workers applied a linear regression analysis to the results of two treadmill tests done two weeks apart in 21 patients in order to quantify the degree of variation occurring (18). They found that a greater than 68% reduction in exercise VPB's must occur before one could be 95% confident that the change was not due to spontaneous variability.

In another study Sami and co-workers analyzed exercise-induced arrhythmia reproducibility in post-myocardial infarction patients (18). A higher degree of reproducibility was found when treadmill tests were performed at relatively short intervals (1 to 2 weeks) than when they were performed at longer intervals (3 to 6 months).

Exercise-induced ventricular arrhythmias manifest at least as much variability as do those detected on ambulatory ECG's. This is true both for both VPB frequency and complexity. Although the data of Faris and co-workers suggest that patients with cardiovascular disease may have a higher degree of reproducibility of exercise-induced arrhythmias, reproducibility in these patients is still low (15).

Factors Influencing Spontaneous Variation

Heart Rate

Several animal studies have observed a relationship between VPB frequency and heart rate (19) and more recently this relationship has been examined in 24 ambulatory patients with frequent VPB's (20). The log of the number of VPB's per 15 minutes was plotted as a function of heart rate. Twenty-three of the patients showed a distinct relationship between VPB frequency and heart rate which was reproducible on a second recording. Twelve patients showed a positive correlation between VPB frequency and heart rate. Seven other patients had a complex relationship. Overall most patients with a complex relationship had most VPB's at higher heart rates. Three patients had relatively flat curves indicating equal numbers of VPB's at each heart rate. One patient had an inverse relationship showing most VPB's at the lowest heart rates. There was no correlation between type of relationship and underlying heart disease.

The predominant pattern of increased VPB frequency with increasing heart rate does not appear to be due to ischemia or simply to the small increases in the number of QRS complexes that occur at higher heart rates. Possible mechanisms for this phenomenon include increased sympathetic activity and/or release of parasympathetic activity at higher heart rates. Calcium channel dependent after-depolarizations are most prominent at higher heart rates and may, in some patients, play a role in the increased ectopy seen at higher heart rates.

Sleep

Sleep has a profound effect on the cardiovascular system, including changes in heart rate, peripheral resistance, blood pressure, and arrhythmias (21, 22). Sleep has an important influence on variation of VPB's that occur throughout the course of a single day. In 1970 Shahaway briefly reported a single patient whose recurrent VT completely and reproducibly disappeared with sleep (23). The most extensive report on the relationship of VPB's to sleep is that of Lown and co-workers (24).

They studied 54 patients who were monitored for 24 hours. Of the 45 patients who had VPB's, the frequency was reduced during sleep in 78% and there was a reduction of 50% or greater in half of the patients. The degree of complexity of the arrhythmias also diminished. In 27% of these patients arrhythmias disappeared entirely during sleep.

Twelve patients with mitral valve prolapse who had frequent VPB's, were analyzed during sleep (25). Seven had a significant reduction in VPB's during sleep, 3 showed no change and 2 showed an increase in VPB's. Of 5 patients with VT, only one had this arrhythmia during sleep (and only on one occasion). Pickering and co-workers analyzed 31 patients with frequent VPB's (26). Eight had complete VPB suppression during sleep, 22 had a lesser reduction, and there was an increase in VPB's in one patient. There have been two studies which have examined the effect of rapid eye movement (REM) sleep with conflicting results. While one study (27) concluded that ventricular irritability increased during REM sleep the other (28) found that there were no changes. Thus it appears that for most patients sleep leads to a decrease in ventricular arrhythmia. A smaller number of patients show no change and a few have an increase in arrhythmias with sleep.

The mechanism by which sleep affects ventricular arrhythmias is not fully defined although changes in autonomic tone, in cardiac work and in heart rate have all been proposed as potential mediators of this effect (29). Changes in heart rate are likely to be one of the most important factors. During sleep there is a fall in heart rate which reaches a nadir after about 6 hours of sleep (17). This diurnal change in heart rate is likely not due to changes in vagal tone, since it has been noted in heart transplant patients and most likely reflects a fall in circulating catecholamines (29). Clearly sleep would explain some of the changes that occur within a day but would generally not explain day-to-day variation.

Degree of Underlying Heart Disease

Calvert and co-workers have performed repeat 24-hour ambulatory ECG monitoring in 65 patients who had had cardiac catheterization and coronary angiography (30). For the group as a whole there was no significant difference in VPB frequency between the two 24-hour monitoring periods. Patients with multivessel coronary disease had significantly ($p<0.02$) more frequent and more complex VPB's than those with single vessel disease or those without heart disease. Severity of heart disease was also a major determinant of reproducibility of severe degrees of arrhythmias. Paired VPB's or VT was reproduced in 40% of those with multivessel disease and in only 29% of those with one or no vessel involvement. Paired VPB's or VT recurred in 60% of those patients with extensive left ventricular asynergy but in none of those without left ventricular asynergy. The authors do not state whether the very mild types of ventricular arrhythmias were more reproducible in those with less severe or no heart disease.

Conclusions

Most studies confirm the fact that there is substantial inherent variability of ventricular arrhythmias both in patients with severe cardiac abnormalities as well as those with more normal hearts. This is true of exercise-induced arrhythmias and of chronic arrhythmias as detected on an ambulatory ECG. Some studies suggest that certain patient subgroups such as those with more severe heart disease (30) or those with very frequent VPB's (6, 8) have more reproducible ventricular arrhythmias. Nonetheless, even these patients manifest a great deal of spontaneous variability of arrhythmias. Although longer periods of monitoring increase the reproducibility from test to test, marked variability exists even between very long recordings (72 hours) (6). One study suggests that month-to-month variability is also an important factor (8).

There are limits to the inherent variability that occurs and because of this ambulatory monitoring and exercise testing can be used to evaluate antiarrhythmic drugs and to predict prognosis. The concept of the inherent variability of ventricular arrhythmias can be incorporated into the design of drug evaluation trials. Large changes in VPB frequency (70–90% reduction) must be demonstrated in individual patients if one is to be confident that a drug is causing a real change. Furthermore, it appears that in patients with low frequency VPB's (less than 2 VPB's/hr) drugs cannot be reliably tested as even a 100% reduction could spontaneously occur reasonably easily (8). Arrhythmias detected on ambulatory monitoring appear to be more reproducible than those induced by exercise and in this respect ambulatory monitoring is the preferred technique for antiarrhythmic drug evaluation (8). Certain patients, however, have their arrhythmia only on exercise and in them exercise testing is of particular value.

When using ambulatory ECG monitoring to predict prognosis one must also be aware of the inherent variability of VPB's. Short monitoring duration may be adequate or even optimal in order to categorize large groups of patients. However, in the case of the individual patient, 24 hours of monitoring may not detect all of those with a specific complex arrhythmia.

There is some evidence that in the post-myocardial infarction patient or chronic coronary artery disease patient the frequency of complex arrhythmias rather than the presence of them places the patient at high risk (12). Consequently a single short period of monitoring may be the most cost-effective means of detecting the high risk patient.

References

1. Myburgh DP, and Van Gelder AL. 1974. The nature of ventricular ectopic beats in chronic ischemic heart disease. South African Medical Journal 48: 1067–1071.
2. Winkle RA. 1978. Antiarrhythmic drug effect mimicked by spontaneous variability of ventricular ectopy. Circulation 57: 1116–1121.

144

3. Kennedy HL, Chandra U, Sayther KL and Caralis DG. 1978. Effectiveness of increasing hours of continuous ambulatory electrocardiography in detecting maximal ventricular ectopy. The American Journal of Cardiology 42: 925–930.

4. Winkle RA, Gradman AH, Fitzgerald JW and Bell PA. 1978. Antiarrhythmic drug efficacy assessed from ventricular arrhythmia reduction in ambulatory electrocardiogram and treadmill test: Comparison of propranolol, procainamide and guinidine. The American Journal of Cardiology 42: 473–480.

5. Pratt CM, Fong A, DeMaria AN, Amsterdam EA and Mason DT. 1979. Recent advances in the understanding of ambulatory electrocardiography. Clinical Cardiology 2: 56–61.

6. Morganroth J, Michelson EL, Horowitz LN, Josephson ME, Pearlman AS and Dunkman WB. 1978. Limitations of routine long-term electrocardiographic monitoring to assess ventricular ectopic beats. Circulation 58: 408–414.

7. Engler R, Ryan W, LeWinter M, Bluestein H and Karliner JS. 1979. Assessment of long-term antiarrhythmic therapy: Studies in the long-term efficacy and toxicity of tocainide. The American Journal of Cardiology 43: 612–618.

8. Sami M, Kraemer H, Harrison DC, Houston N, Shunasaki C and DeBusk RF. 1980. A new method for evaluating antiarrhythmic drug efficacy. Circulation 62: 1172–1179.

9. Ruberman W, Weinblatt E, Goldberg JD, Frank CW and Shapiro S. 1977. Ventricular premature beats and mortality after myocardial infarction. New England Journal of Medicine 297: 750–757.

10. Michelson EL and Morganroth J. 1980. Spontaneous variability of complex ventricular arrhythmias detected by long-term electrocardiographic recording. Circulation 61: 690–695.

11. Thanavaro S, Kleiger RE, Hieb BR, Krone RJ, deMello VR and Oliver GC. 1980. Effect of electrocardiographic recording duration on ventricular dysrhythmic detection after myocardial infarction. Circulation 62: 262–265.

12. Winkle RA, Peters F and Hall R. 1981. Characterization of ventricular tachyarrhythmias on ambulatory ECG recordings in post-myocardial infarction patients: Arrhythmia detection and duration of recording, relationship between arrhythmia frequency and complexity, and day-to-day reproducibility. American Heart Journal 102: 162–169.

13. Astrand I. 1965. Exercise electrocardiogram recorded twice with an 8-year interval in a group of 204 women and men 48–63 years old. Acta Medica Scandinavica 178: 27–39.

14. Jelinek MV and Lown B. 1974. Exercise stress testing for exposure of cardiac arrhythmia. Progress in Cardiovascular Diseases 16: 497–522.

15. Faris JV, McHenry PL, Jordan JW and Morris SN. 1976. Prevalence and reproducibility of exercise-induced ventricular arrhythmias during maximal exercise testing in normal men. The American Journal of Cardiology 37: 617–622.

16. DeBaker G, Jacobs D, Prineas R, Crow R, Vilandre J and Blackburn H. 1978. Ventricular premature beats. Cardiology 63: 53–63.

17. Sheps DL, Ernst JC, Briese FR, Lopez LU, Conde CA, Castellanos A and Meyerburg RJ. 1977. Decreases frequency of exercise-induced ventricular ectopic activity in the second of two consecutive treadmill tests. Circulation 55: 892–895.

18. Sami M, Kraemer H and DeBusk RF. 1979. Reproducibility of exercise-induced ventricular arrhythmia after myocardial infarction. The American Journal of Cardiology 43: 724–730.

19. Han J, DeFragha J, Millet D and Moe GK. 1966. Incidence of ectopic beats as a function of basic rate in the ventricle. American Heart Journal 72: 632–639.

20. Winkle RA. The relationship between ventricular ectopic beat frequency and heart rate. (In press).

21. Tzivoni D and Stern S. 1973. Electrocardiographic pattern during sleep in healthy subjects and in patients with ischemic heart disease. Journal of Electrocardiography 6: 225–229.

22. Khatri IM and Freis ED. 1967. Hemodynamic changes during sleep. Journal of Applied

145

Physiology 22: 867–873.
23. Shahaway ME. 1970. Arrhythmias and the varieties of sleep (letter). New England Journal of Medicine 282: 815.
24. Lown B, Tykocinski M, Garfein A and Brooks P. 1973. Sleep and ventricular premature beats. Circulation 48: 691–701.
25. Winkle RA, Lopes MG, Fitzgerald JW, Goodman DJ, Schroeder JS, and Harrison DC. 1975. Arrhythmias in patients with mitral valve prolapse. Circulation 52: 73–81.
26. Pickering TG, Goulding L and Cobern BA. 1977. Diurnal variations in ventricular ectopic beats and heart rate. Cardiovascular Medicine 2: 1013.
27. Rosenblatt G, Hartmann E and Zwilling GR. 1973. Cardiac irritability during sleep and dreaming. Journal of Psychosomatic Research 17: 129–134.
28. Smith R, Johnson L, Rothfield D, Zir L and Tharp B. 1972. Sleep and cardiac arrhythmias. Archives of Internal Medicine 130: 751–753.
29. Winkle RA. 1978. "Circadian variations in ventricular ectopic activity," in Management of Ventricular Tachycardia – Role of Mexilitine. Edited by Sandøe E, Julian DG and Bell JW. Excerpta Medica, pg. 165–169.
30. Calvert A, Lown B and Gorlin R. 1977. Ventricular premature beats and anatomically defined coronary artery disease. The American Journal of Cardiology 39: 627–634.

CLASSIFICATION OF CARDIAC ARRHYTHMIAS AND CONDUCTION DEFECTS FOR RISK ASSESSMENT

H.E. KULBERTUS

1. Characterization of Ventricular Extrasystoles after Myocardial Infarction

Approximately 10% of the patients having suffered a myocardial infarction die during the first year following their acute illness. Several studies have investigated the role of Holter ambulatory monitoring in the identification of patients at increased risk of sudden death: conflicting results have been reported.

Obviously, the major problem one encounters in trying to understand the differences between the results lies in the lack of a homogenous classification of the arrhythmias.

1.1. Lown's Grading System

The most frequently quoted grading system is that proposed by Lown and Wolf in 1971 (1). Table 1 gives the definitions for the Lown's grades. The system is mutually exclusive and hierarchical: grades are assigned on the basis of the highest grade recorded.

Table 1. The Lown's grading system for ventricular arrhythmias (1).

Lown's grade	Definition
0	No ventricular premature beat
1	Less than 30 ventricular premature beats per hour
2	30 or more ventricular premature beats per hour
3	Multiform ventricular extrasystoles
4a	Two consecutive ventricular premature beats
4b	Three or more consecutive ventricular premature beats
5	R on T (RV/QT less than 1.0)
Grades are assigned on the basis of the highest ranking characteristic	

The underlying assumption is that the hierarchy of Lown's grades parallels the hierarchy of risk. For instance, if a patient shows R-on-T ventricular premature beats, this feature is considered to be of such ominous significance that the concomitant presence of multiform ventricular extrasystoles may be disregarded.

For the analysis of 24-hour tapes, Lown et al (2) have developed a more complex expression which indicates the number of hours during which a particular grade has been achieved. This is marked by exponents. Subscripts are used for defining particular aspects of ventricular ectopic activity.

A subscript for grade 2 indicates the approximate total number of VPB's per 24 hour. For grade 3, it denotes the number of foci observed. For grade 4 (a), the subscript indicates the maximum number of couplets seen in any single hour. For grade 4 (b), two subscripts separated by a dash are used: the first indicates the number of paroxysms of tachycardia and the second the largest number of successive cycles. For grade 5, the subscript presents the largest number of R-on-T premature beats in any single hour.

Thus $0^4 \; 1^3 \; 2^6_{840} \; 3^6_2 \; 4\,(a)^2_3 \; 4\,(b)^2_{3\text{-}6} \; 5^1_2$ should read as follows:

1) There were 4 hours free of VPB activity
2) During 3 hours, the grade reached was 1
3) During 6 hours, the grade reached was 2 and the approximate total number of VPB's was 840.
4) Multifocal VPB's were seen during 6 hours and 2 different foci were noted.
5) Couplets were observed in 2 monitored hours and the largest number of couplets in one single hour was 3.
6) Episodes of ventricular tachycardia were noted in two of the monitored hours (three paroxysms, the longest of 6 successive cycles).
7) An R-on-T phenomenon was noted on two occasions during one of the monitored hours.

This notation system surely deserved interest: however, it is not yet widely known and has apparently never been used for observational studies in ischemic heart disease.

1.2. Classification of Ventricular Arrhythmias in Published Post Myocardial Infarction Studies

In the recent past, a number of follow-up investigations (3 to 11) have examined the role of Holter monitoring for identifying post myocardial infarction patients at high risk of subsequent death. These studies have generally shown a correlation between asymptomatic ventricular arrhythmias and subsequent untoward effects.

A detailed analysis of studies published before 1979 was made by Winkle (12). This author pointed out that different definitions of complex arrhythmias were used by different investigators and that, in some instances, bigeminy, R-on-T or multifocality were not even considered. Most studies included data on VPB's frequency, but they generally used one single partition value which leads to a considerably loss of information. The frequency of occurrence of complex arrhythmias was generally not included in the analysis of risk. Most investigators used an arbitrary classification derived from Lown's and only recorded the highest grade reached; this approach ignores the possible significance of lesser grades of arrhythmias. The same holds true for those who combined several grades of arrhythmias in the final data analysis (for example, simple versus complex arrhythmias). Finally, the studies varied considerably in terms of duration of electrocardiographic monitoring (ranging from 1 to 24 hours) and in terms of delay between time of Holter monitoring and time of infarction.

Winkle (12) quite righteously noted "that most of the studies showing the prognostic value of arrhythmias on ambulatory recordings in the late post myocardial infarction period utilized recordings of less than 12 hours' duration". Only one (12) of the studies using 24 hour recordings found a relationship between ventricular arrhythmias and subsequent deaths. This may reflect that after 24 hours of recording, the great majority (+ 80%) of post myocardial infarction patients are found to have some form of complex arrhythmias. This finding becomes too frequent and therefore looses its clinical usefulness.

1.3. More Recent Studies

Ruberman et al (13) recently completed a study of 1739 male survivors of myocardial infarction who had a 1 hour single lead electrocardiographic recording on tape. Half of the patients had a myocardial infarction within 3 months before examination, an additional 30% within 3–8 months and 20% had had silent myocardial infarcts or intervals of at least 9 months since the last acute episode. Complex ventricular arrhythmias consisted of R-on-T, runs of 2 or more, multiform or bigeminal complexes. At 5 years, the cumulative probability of sudden death (age-adjusted) in the men who had such arrhythmias was 18% compared with 8% in others. Among those who had runs or R-on-T complexes, the age-adjusted probability of sudden death at 5 years was 25%, compared with 13% among men with other forms of complex VPB's, 12% among those with simple VPB's and 6% among those without VPB's during the monitored hour. R-on-T beats or runs were thus the features which best identified patients at very high risk of sudden death; this suggests that such ectopic forms are uniquely related to ventricular fibrillation as opposed to congestive heart failure which had a stronger influence on risk of other types of cardiac deaths.

Bigger et al (14), in an excellent recent study, discussed the short-comings of Lown's grading system which they tested in a group of 400 patients having recently experienced an acute myocardial infarction. They showed that the death rate (mean follow-up of 30 months) did not steadily increase as a function of Lown's arrhythmic grade, but that the mortality rate was significantly higher in grades 4 b (three or more consecutive ventricular extrasystoles) and 5 (R-on-T phenomenon) than in the other five grades (p < 0.01).

Their second conclusion was that there existed a progressive rise in mortality rate with increasing frequency of ventricular premature beats. Therefore, the practice of using a single partition value of VPB's frequency, to assign risk would always ignore much valuable information. In their series, there was a strong association between high frequency and complexity of ventricular extrasystoles. Nevertheless, the frequency of VPB's continued to exert an adverse influence even in persons who had complex ventricular extrasystolic features.

Finally, they observed a great heterogeneity of outcome among the subgroups which make up one of Lown's grade. For example, patients in grade 5 with low VPB's frequency and no complex feature except R-on-T had a very low mortality rate (9%) whereas those with a high frequency of VPB's and all complex features had a very high mortality rate (59%).

In another recent paper, Winkle et al (15) demonstrated that if one repeats 24 hour Holter monitoring on several consecutive days, there is a remarkable increase in the detection of specific types of complex VPB's for recording periods beyond 24 hours. The same authors also indicated that patients whose complex VPB's were detected with shorter durations of monitoring were those who had these arrhythmias present during the highest percentage of the time. Once again, they stressed that it may be the frequency of complex arrhythmias which places the patients at high risk rather than merely the presence or absence of these arrhythmias. Should this be true, single short recording periods might be preferable for screening rather than longer and more quantitatively characterized ambulatory electrocardiographic recordings which might become too sensitive. Winkle et al (15) finally insisted on the fact that complex forms may, at times, be present in patients with very unfrequent VPB's.

1.4. Which Classification Should Be Recommended?

It may appear disappointing that, while so many studies have been devoted to this problem, no satisfactory classification of ventricular arrhythmias following myocardial infarction has been achieved as yet.

On the whole, it is generally agreed that a strong correlation exists between ventricular arrhythmias observed on Holter recordings and subsequent sudden death in post myocardial infarction patients. Frequent VPB's, repetitive extrasystoles and VPB's showing the R-on-T phenomenon seem to carry the most ominous prognostic significance.

It would probably be useless to propose one single classification for ventricular arrhythmias after myocardial infarction. Indeed, the choice must be guided by the reason why risk stratification is attempted.

If one wishes, for examples, to exclude a very low risk subset from some form of treatment, the criteria of less than 1 VPB per hour may be suggested (14). On the opposite, if one wishes to select the patients at highest risk, for intervention studies, then it might be justified to select those with frequent VPB's (>30/hour) associated with either repetitive responses or premature extrasystoles showing the R-on-T phenomenon.

One should be aware that, at present, such criteria may be used to select subsets of individuals with a given risk; they do not however allow conclusions regarding the prognosis of each individual patient.

There is still a need for further studies based on carefully analyzed and quantified ambulatory electrocardiographic recordings performed over long periods of time (72 hours would be my proposal since the cumulative number of patients with each type of complex VPB's appears to be at or near a plateau by the end of the 72 hour recording period (15)). The 72 hour recordings should be repeated at various moments during the first three months following the acute myocardial infarction. Then, by using sophisticated statistical methods of discriminant analysis one should be able to determine which is the most appropriate timing and the most effective duration of Holter monitoring for risk stratification after myocardial infarction. A simple index based on the frequency of occurrence of various complex VPB's would be derived. It would be applicable to the individual patient and might help in therapeutic decision making.

2. Ventricular Premature Beats in Individuals Without Ischemic Heart Disease

The prognostic significance of complex VPB's is established only when they occur after myocardial infarction. In this setting, although the data are somewhat conflicting, it appears that there exists a relationship between their occurrence and either the number of vessels diseased or the degree of left ventricular dysfunction (12).

It has been suggested, however, that if ambulatory recordings are made long after the acute myocardial infarction, ventricular arrhythmias might lose their prognostic significance (7). What is then their meaning in patients without overt ischemic heart disease?

In their study of employed males aged 35 to 65, Hinkle et al. (16) found an increased prevalence of VPB's with increasing age. Complex VPB's occurred more frequently in subjects with frequent VPB's. Frequent VPB's ($>10/10.000$) primarily occurred in individuals with evidence of cardiac disease and were associated with an increased risk of coronary death or sudden cardiac death. The most interesting conclusion of this study was that, in the absence of coronary disease or risk factors, frequent VPB's did not seem to predict subsequent death.

Complex ventricular arrhythmias are not a rare finding in 24 hour recordings (17) of apparently healthy individuals (Table 2).

Multifocal VPB's occur quite frequently (up to 10–15% in some studies). Pairs, bigeminal rhythm and ventricular tachycardia are much less common.

Ventricular tachycardia during ambulatory recording has been reported in at least 4 "healthy" individuals. Brodsky et al (18) reported an episode with 5 con-

Table 2. Prevalence of complex VPB's in 260 healthy individuals, studied by 24 hour ambulatory electrocardiographic recording. (The numbers indicate % of subjects studied). From Bjerregaard P (17).

	Age (yrs)			
	40–49	50–59	60–79	All
Multifocal VPB's	12	22	19	20
Paired VPB's	3	9	8	8
Coupled VPB's	2	1	1	2
Ventricular tachycardia	3	1	1	2

secutive VPB's at a rate of 136/min occurring during sleep in a subject who had no other VPB in his 24-hour recording. Djiane et al (19) observed a similar episode of ventricular tachycardia occurring during sleep. Clarke et al (20) noted an episode of ventricular tachycardia during sleep and one during the day in 2 women who had no other complex ventricular arrhythmia in their Holter recordings.

The problem of determining whether VPB's or other arrhythmias provide a significant independent contribution to prognosis in apparently healthy people remains unsettled.

Multivariate analysis studies indicate that arrhythmias covary with various risk factors for coronary artery disease (for example, age and hypertension (17). As yet, a clearcut independent prognostic contribution of arrhythmias has not been defined in asymptomatic individuals.

3. Conduction Disorders Observed on Holter Monitoring

3.1. S-A Block and Sinus Pauses

Short sinus pauses (average duration: 1.2 sec) are frequent and were observed in 49% of normal individuals studied by Engel and Burckhardt (21). Sinus pauses in excess of 2 seconds constitute a very unusual finding in healthy subjects (Table 3).

Pauses of 2 seconds or more are therefore considered by some as a criterion for established sinus node disease (22).

The prognostic significance of sinus node disease remains incompletely kown. Rasmussen (23) has studied 24 patients followed up without pacing for an average of 7 years. During this follow-up no death was noted. In view of this, Rasmussen advocates that, regardless of the duration of the pauses, one should insert a pacemaker only when the patients' symptoms clearly indicate the need for it.

Table 3. Longest sinus pauses during 24 hour ambulatory electrocardiographic recordings in healthy subjects. (The numbers indicate % of subjects studied). From Bjerregaard P. (17)

Authors	> 1500 msec	> 1750 msec	> 2000 msec
Brodsky et al (18) (age 23–27 yrs)	68	28	4
Djiane et al (19) (age 32 ± 9 yrs)	48	12	4
Bjerregaard (17)			
Age 40–49 yrs	37	3	1
Age 50–59 yrs	31	3	1
Age 60–79 yrs	19	7	0

3.2. Atrioventricular Block

Aggravation of first degree A-V block and development of Wenckebach AV block during phases of parasympathetic overactivity have been demonstrated in healthy subjects (17). Wenckebach AV block is a frequent feature following heavy physical training (24). It may also be observed in so-called normal subjects during sleep (20).

Intermittent complete AV block has never been reported during ambulatory electrocardiographic monitoring of healthy subjects. Our impression is that Mobitz type II 2nd degree and 3rd degree AV blocks always represent abnormal findings and deserve special attention. However, subsamples of AV node disease such as congenital heart block or proximal complete block may have a good prognosis and be followed for years without deterioration or even need for pacemaker implantation.

3.3. Bundle Branch Block

Patients with bundle branch block or incomplete bilateral bundle branch block (right bundle block with left fascicular block) are generally considered as being at risk of developing complete heart block or sudden death (by asystole or, probably, more often, ventricular fibrillation).

The risk is strongly influenced by the characteristics of the population from which the patients are derived.

In a recent study, electrocardiograms (25) were recorded on 30,001 ambulatory individuals submitted to a screening programme for hypertension. Among the 129 instances of RBBB-LAHB, the cumulative mortality at 4 years was 18.6% and the cumulative mortality from cardiac death 7%. The risk of developing complete heart block was 8% at 5 years.

These findings contrast with the data reported from Portland where Mc Anulty et al (26) studied a large hospital based series. In their experience, patients with RBBB-LAHB had a much higher death rate (49% at 5 years). Their series however contained a large proportion of patients with known cardiovascular disease.

In spite of these differences of outcome in relation to the clinical conditions, every one agrees that patients with these conduction disturbances should be paced when they are asymptomatic or when they show episodes of Mobitz type II 2nd degree or 3rd degree AV block on their Holter monitoring.

The long term prognostic significance of bundle branch block complicating acute myocardial infarction remains a subject of debate. An important multicentre study involving 432 patients with infarction and bundle branch block was reported in 1978 (27). Patients who had developed transient high degree AV block during infarction had a 28% rate of sudden death or recurrent high degree AV block in the first year of follow-up. This contrasts with the figure of 13% obtained among those who did not develop this complication. Of the 14 sudden deaths or episodes of recurrent high degree AV block which occurred in patients who had progressed to high degree AV block while hospitalized, 3 occurred in the group of 30 patients discharged with a permanent pacemaker (10%) whereas 11 sudden deaths or episodes of high degree block occurred in the group of 20 patients discharged without permanent pacemaker (55%; p < 0.01). Careful monitoring of AV conduction is therefore mandatory in patients with acute myocardial infarction and bundle branch block and permanent pacing is indicated in those who, at some time of their illness, progress to high degree AV block.

References

1. Lown B, Wolf M, 1971. Approach to sudden death from coronary heart disease. Circulation, 44 – 130–42.
2. Lown B, Calvert AF, Armington R, Ryan M, 1975. Monitoring for serious arrhythmias and high risk of sudden death. Circulation, suppl III, 51–52, 189–198.
3. Bigger JT, Heller CA, Wenger TL, Weld FM, 1978. Risk stratification after acute myocardial infarction. Amer J Cardiol, 42, 202–210.
4. De Busk RF, Davidson DM, Houston N, Fitzgerald JW. 1980. Serial ambulatory electrocardiography and treadmill exercise testing following uncomplicated myocardial infarction. Amer J Cardiol, 45, 547.
5. Kotler MN, Tabatznik B, Mower MM, Tominaga, S., 1973. Prognostic significance of ventricular ectopic beats with respect to sudden death in the late post-infarction period. Circulation, 47, 959.
6. Luria MH, Knoke JD, Margolis RM, Hendricks FH, Kublic B., 1976. Acute myocardial infarction: prognosis after recovery. Ann Intern Med 85, 561.
7. Moss AJ, Davis HT, De Camilla J, Bayer LW, 1979. Ventricular ectopic beats and their relation to sudden and non-sudden cardiac death after myocardial infarction. Circulation 60, 998.
8. Rehnqvist N, Sjogren A. 1977. Ventricular arrhythmias prior to discharge and one year after acute myocardial infarction. Europ J Cardiol, 575, 425.
9. Ruberman W, Weinblatt E, Goldberg J, Frank CW, Shapiro S, 1977. Ventricular premature beats and mortality after myocardial infarction. N Engl J Med 297, 750.
10. Schulze RA Jr, Strauss HW, Pitt B. 1977. Sudden death in the year following myocardial infarction. Amer J Med 62, 192.
11. Vismara LA, Amsterdam EA, Mason DT, 1975. Relation of ventricular arrhythmias in

the late hospital phase of acute myocardial infarction to sudden death after hospital discharge. Am J Med 59, 6.

12. Winkle RA. 1980. Detection of patients at high risk for sudden death: the role of electrocardiographic monitoring. p. 275 in Sudden Death. Kulbertus HE and Wellens HJJ editors, Martinus Nijhoff, The Hague.

13. Ruberman W, Weinblatt E, Goldberg JD, Frank ChW, Chaudary BS, Shapiro. 1981. Ventricular premature complexes and sudden death after myocardial infarction. Circulation 64, 297–305.

14. Bigger J Th, Weld FM, 1981. Analysis of prognostic significance of ventricular arrhythmias after myocardial infarction. Shortcomings of Lown grading system. Brit Heart J 45, 717–724.

15. Winkle RA, Peters Fl, Hall R. 1981. Characterization of ventricular tachyarrhythmias on ambulatory ECG recordings in post-myocardial infarction patients: arrhythmia detection and duration of recordings, relationship between arrhythmia frequency and complexity, and day-to-day reproducibility. Am Heart J 102, 162–169.

16. Hinkle LE, Carver ST, Agyros DC, 1975. The prognostic significance of ventricular premature beats in healthy people and in people with coronary artery disease. Acta Cardiologica (suppl.) 18, 5.

17. Bjerregaard P. 1980. Prevalence and variability of cardiac arrhythmias in healthy subjects. in Cardiac arrhythmias in the active population. p 24–32. Chamberlain D, Kulbertus HE, Mogensen L and Schlepper M. Ed. AB Hässle, Mölndal.

18. Brodsky M, Wu D, Denes P, Kanakis C, Rosen KM. 1977. Arrhythmia documented by 24 hour continuous electrocardiographic monitoring in 50 male medical students without apparent heart disease. Am J Cardiol 39, 390–395.

19. Djiane P, Egre A, Bory M, Savin B, Serradimigni A. 1977. L'enregistrement électrocardiographique continu chez 50 sujets normaux. in Troubles du rythme et électrostimulation p. 161–168. Puel P. Ed. Nouvelle Imprimerie Fournié. Toulouse.

20. Clarke J.M, Hamer J, Shelton JR, Taylor S, Venning GR. 1976, The Rhythm of the normal human heart. Lancet 2, 508–512.

21. Engel UR, Burckhardt D. 1975. Haüfigkeit und Art von Herzrhythmusstörungen sowie EKG. Schweiz Med Wochenschr 105, 1467–1469.

22. Shaw DB. 1980. The incidence and prevalence of bradyarrhythmias in Cardiac arrhythmias in the active population. p. 35–37. Chamberlain D, Kulbertus HE, Mogensen L, Schlepper M, Eds. AB Hässle. Mölndal.

23. Rasmussen K 1971. Chronic sino-atrial block. Amer Heart J, 81, 39–47.

24. Meytes Kaplinsky E, Yahini JH, Hanne-Papporo N, Neufeld HN. 1975. Wenckebach AV block: A frequent feature following heavy physical training. Am Heart J, 90, 426–430.

25. Kulbertus HE, de Leval-Rutten F, Dubois M, Petit JM. 1980. Sudden death in subjects with intraventricular conduction detects. in Sudden death. p 379–391. Kulbertus HE and Wellens HJJ Eds. Martinus Nijhoff, The Hague.

26. Mc Anulty JH, Rahimtoola SH, Murphy ES, Kauffman S, Ritzmann LW, Kanarek P, Demots H. 1978. A prospective study of sudden death in "high risk" bundle branch block. New England J of Med, 299, 209–215.

27. Hindman MC, Wagner GS, Jaro M, Atkins JM, Scheinman MM, De Sanctis RW, Hutter AH, Yeatman L, Rubenfire M, Pujura C, Rubin M, Morris JJ. 1978. The clinical significance of bundle branch block complicating acute myocardial infarction. 2. Indication for temporary and permanent pacemaker insertion. Circulation 58, 689–699.

PROGNOSTIC ASPECTS OF VENTRICULAR ARRHYTHMIAS IN PATIENTS WITH CORONARY ARTERY DISEASE*

A.J. MOSS, M.D.

1. Introduction

Ventricular premature beats (VPBs) are omnipresent in the general population, but their occurrence in patients with coronary artery disease warrants special consideration. Interest in VPBs has increased in the past decade because of: 1) the well-documented relationship between VPBs and ventricular fibrillation in acute myocardial infarction; 2) numerous studies substantiating a strong association between VPBs and sudden cardiac death in sub-acute and chronic coronary disease; 3) improved techniques for identifying VPBs utilizing telemetry and Holter methods; and 4) the potential for "preventing" VPB-induced ventricular fibrillation events.

The prognostic aspects of ventricular premature beats will be related to the occurrence of ventricular arrhythmias occurring in the post-hospital phase of myocardial infarction. Only those ventricular arrhythmias identified on ambulatory Holter recordings in this specific population will be reviewed.

2. Classification of VPBs

Numerous schemes have been used to classify Holter recorded VPBs. Ruberman (1) and Moss (2) have categorized VPBs into complex and simple groupings. Complex VPBs include those with multiform configuration, repetitive beating, early cycle complexes ($RR'/QT \leqslant 1.00$), or bigeminal rhythm. Simple VPBs are those that do not have any of the above complex configurations. The more widely used Lown (3) grading system utilizes a five-level, mutually exclusive, hierarchical schema with grades assigned on the basis of the highest ranking characteristic. Recently, Bigger (4) has pointed out the shortcomings of the Lown grading system particularly as it relates to non-overlapping of risk and the low weight assigned

* Supported in part by NHLBI grants HL-15790 and HL-22982 and by the Gebbie Foundation, Jamestown, New York.

to frequent VPBs. Bigger showed that VPB frequency bears a direct relationship to mortality that repetitive VPBs carry an independent risk, and the highest risk occurrs in patients with frequent and repetitive VPBs. Early cycle R-on-T VPBs did not contribute independent risk. It is clear that a great deal more work needs to be done in the prognostic classification of VPBs.

3. VPBs and Multifactorial Risk

In our previously reported Rochester Heart Research Follow-up Study (5) we prospectively studied 978 post-infarction patients with predischarge six-hour Holter recordings and followed the outcome of these patients for periods ranging from two to four years. All patients had a documented acute myocardial infarction and were less than 66 years of age. The average age was 53.7 years and 81% were men. During follow-up there were 136 total deaths with 117 cardiac deaths. Univariate analysis demonstrated that the following factors were associated with a significantly ($P < 0.01$) increased occurrence of cardiac death: prior myocardial infarction, left ventricular dysfunction in the coronary care unit, anterior myocardial infarction, and one or more VPBs on the predischarge Holter. Multivariate survivorship analysis demonstrated that the highest mortality risk occurred in those patients with a combination of anterior myocardial infarction, left ventricular dysfunction and one or more VPBs. In contrast, an extremely low-risk group with a four-year survival of 96% occurred in patients who had none of the following: prior myocardial infarction before the index coronary event, left ventricular dysfunction, or VPBs. (Table 1).

Table 1. Multivariate survival during the posthospital phase of myocardial infarction.

Risk Group	Percent of Population	Characteristics*	Survival	
			6 months	24 months
Low	24%	NO PMI, LVD, or VPB	98%	96%
Intermediate	61%	NON LO/HI	93%	88%
High	15%	AMI + LVD + VPB	86%	77%

* PMI = prior myocardial infarction; LVD = left ventricular dysfunction; VPB = ventricular premature beats; AMI = anterior myocardial infarction.

4. Sudden Cardiac Death

We investigated the relationship between VPBs and sudden and non-sudden cardiac death using the one-hour definition for sudden. A strong association exists between the occurrence of complex VPBs on the predischarge Holter recording and the subsequent occurrence of both sudden and non-sudden cardiac death. There was a progressive gradient in mortality, both sudden and non-sudden cardiac death, among patients with none, simple, and complex VPBs (Table 2). Recently, Kleiger and associates (5) investigated the relationship between the percent risk of ventricular runs (repetitive VPBs) and sudden death after myocardial infarction. They identified patients according to the quartile of risk of having ventricular runs. The patients with the highest probability of having ventricular runs had a mortality rate that was no different than those who had the lowest probability of having ventricular runs. They concluded that the presence of ventricular runs in their population seemed to be a marker of severe cardiac disease rather than an independent factor for an increased incidence of sudden death.

Table 2. Predischarge Holter VPB categories and the occurrence of sudden and non-sudden cardiac death during the posthospital phase of myocardial infarction.

Holter	Cardiac death (%)			
VPBs	1 YEAR		3 YEARS	
	Sudden	Non-sudden	Sudden	Non-sudden
NONE	1.8	1.5	3.9	2.8
SIMPLE	3.8	1.8	6.1	5.0
COMPLEX	6.8	7.5	13.5	9.8

* COMPLEX VPBs = multiform configuration, repetitive beating, early cycle complexes RR'/ QT ⩽1.00), or bigeminal rhythm. SIMPLE VPBs = those with non-complex configuration.

5. Ventricular Tachycardia

During the course of the Holter monitoring of our post-infarction population before discharge and at four-month intervals thereafter, we identified 66 patients with one or more episodes of ventricular tachycardia. A double set of controls (n=132) without ventricular tachycardia was matched by gender, date of entry, and date of follow-up Holter recording to the 66 patients with ventricular tachycardia. Despite the matching, the ventricular tachycardia patients had a significantly higher Peel score (7) and more frequent VPBs on the Holter recording. Life table analysis of the survival of ventricular tachycardia and control patients revealed a 48-months survival of 75% and 87%, respectively (8). The risk of ventricular tachycardia patients dying was 2.35 (95% confidence interval 0.82% to 6.77) times that of patients without ventricular tachycardia. Among those who died, the age, sex, cause of death, suddenness of death, and mechanism of death were similar in the ventricular tachycardia and control patients. Within the tachycardia group, those who died had more severe underlying heart disease then the survivors. The occurrence of ventricular tachycardia in the post-hospital phase of myocardial infarction, while associated with a somewhat lower survival rate, does not indicate as much danger as generally assumed.

6. The Interaction of Digitals and VPBs

The effect of digitalis (digoxin) therapy on a four-month post-hospital cardiac mortality was investigated in 812 patients who survived the hospital phase of acute myocardial infarction (9). A step wise multiple logistic regression analysis was utilized to identify variables associated with increased mortality and to adjust for differences in confounding variables between digitalis and non-digitalis patients. The major four-month mortality (38.5%) occurred in digitalis-treated patients with congestive heart failure during the CCU and complex VPBs on a predischarge Holter recording. Logistic analyses which controlled for confounding variables indicated that digitalis use contributed to the increased mortality rate in this high-risk subset. This retrospective study suggests that digitalis use increases early post-hospital mortality of myocardial infarction patients with combined electrical and mechanical dysfunction. This retrospective analysis of the data from our Heart Research Follow-Up Study has definite limitation since statistical adjustment techniques were required to control for the severity of the underlying cardiac disease in those patients with and without digitalis therapy. A prospective digitalis withdrawal trial is needed to definitively answer the question of the role of digitalis in enhancing post-infarction mortality. However, the retrospective analysis does highlight the importance of the interaction of factors (complex VPBs, left ventricular dysfunction, and digitalis therapy) in affecting outcome.

7. Conclusion

Studies from our laboratory and by other investigators in the field indicate that the presence of ventricular arrhythmias in patients with coronary artery disease is related to the extent and severity of active myocardial ischemia, the degree of myocardial-left ventricular dysfunction, and to certain neurogenic factors involving the central and sympathetic nervous system. The independent contribution of ventricular arrhythmias to cardiac mortality is difficult to substantiate. At the present time, the prognostic significance of VPBs involves a complex interaction with ischemic mechanical, neurogenic, and drug related factors. From the available data, "complex" VPBs are surely a marker of a high-risk individual, and in selected patients, frequent and repetitive VPBs may be a primary trigger of ventricular fibrillation.

References

1. Ruberman W, Weinblatt E, Goldberg J, Frank C, Shapiro S: Ventricular premature beats and mortality after myocardial infarction. New Engl J Med 297: 750, 1977.
2. Moss A, Davis H, DeCamilla J, Bayer L: Ventricular ectopic beats and their relation to sudden and non-sudden cardiac death after myocardial infarction. Circulation 60:

998, 1979.

3. Lown B, Wolf M: Approaches to sudden death from coronary heart disease. Circulation 44: 130, 1971.

4. Bigger JT Jr, Weld F: Analysis of prognostic significance of ventricular arrhythmias after myocardial infarction. Brit Med J 45: 717, 1981.

5. Davis H, DeCamilla J, Bayer L, Moss A: Survivorship patterns in the posthospital phase of myocardial infarction. Circulation 60: 1252, 1979.

6. Kleiger R, Miller P, Thanavaro S, Province M, Martin T, Oliver C: Relationship between clinical features of acute myocardial infarction and ventricular runs at 2 weeks and 1 year after infarction. Circulation 63: 64, 1981.

7. Peel A, Semple T, Wang I, Lancaster W, Dall J: A coronary prognostic index for grading the severity of infarction. Brit Heart J 24: 745, 1962.

8. Anderson K, DeCamilla J, Moss A: Clinical significance of ventricular tachycardia detected during ambulatory monitoring after myocardial infarction. Circulation 57: 890, 1978.

9. Moss A, Davis H, Conard D, DeCamilla J, Odoroff C: Digitalis associated cardiac mortality after myocardial infarction. Circulation 64 (in press) 1981.

DESIGN OF SECONDARY PREVENTIVE TRIALS WITH ANTI-ARRHYTHMIC AGENTS: THE RIGHT QUESTION WITH THE WRONG ANSWER

J. LUBSEN*

Introduction

Sudden cardiac death (SD) due to ventricular fibrillation (VF) remains one of the enigmas of contemporary cardiology. In a considerable fraction of all deaths from Coronary Heart Disease (CHD), it is the first clinical manifestation of the disease. In patients who cross the clinical horizon of CHD otherwise, by the development of angina or acute myocardial infarction for instance, SD due to VF is the most feared future complication. Therefore, prevention of SD is one, if not the primary, objective of secondary preventive measures in patients with established CHD.

As secondary preventive measure especially aimed to prevent SD, anti-arrhythmic treatment has found strong advocates. (1) To argue their case, they point out that ventricular arrhythmias are a potent risk-indicator in patients with coronary heart disease, that electrically unstable ventricles fibrillate and that anti-arrhythmic agents stabilize the ventricle, thereby suppressing arrhythmias and, presumably, VF. Furthermore, they argue that comparatively simple methods to detect ventricular arrhythmias as evidence of (tendency to) electrical unstability are now available, notably 24-hour ambulatory ECG monitoring. Patients with CHD and ventricular arrhythmias are then obvious candidates for anti-arrhythmic treatment. Today, many such patients receive this treatment, not so much because the arrhythmia causes any discomfort but because it is assumed that the risk of fatal VF is thereby reduced. However reasonable the rationale which supports any drug treatment, it is now generally accepted that clinical trials are needed to establish efficacy before a treatment recommendation can be made. The need to do clinical trials is particularly strong when a form of therapy is proposed of which the harmful effects may outweigh the benefits, as is often the case when potent drugs are used for prolonged periods of time, for instance in secondary prevention of CHD. As discussed by Dr. van Durme, (2) secondary preventive trials with antiarrhythmic agents have indeed been done. So far, they have not

* Thoraxcenter, Rotterdam.

shown any beneficial effect. There may be many reasons for this apparent failure. One may be that anti-arrhythmic agents in fact do not prevent VF. Another may be that the studies done so far have simply been to small and/or to inefficient in the selection of really suitable study subjects, i.e. patients at a particular high risk of VF. Finally, the design of the studies done may have been inappropriate. It is the purpose of this presentation to elaborate further on this last possibility. Results from the Ghent Rotterdam Aprindine (GRAP) Study (2) will be used as an example and an alternative approach to design of arrhythmia trials will be discussed, with particular attention to the possible role of 24-hour ECG monitoring.

As an Example: Results of a Particular Trial

The design of the GRAP study has been extensively described elsewhere. (3) From the design point-of-view, the study follows a classical pattern. Patients in whom the indication for a particular treatment are thought to exist, are randomized to either active drug or placebo. In the GRAP-study, the indication was "status post-MI, with complex ventricular arrhythmias on a 24-hour ECG (defined as *either* more than 5 premature ventricular complexes (PVCs) in any minute of recording *or* multiform PVCs *or* runs of two or more PVCs)". A total of 300 patients in whom this indication was established were included.

The study treatment was the anti-arrhythmic agent aprindine: 151 patients were randomized to receive active drug and 149 to placebo. A special feature was the method of dose adjustment. The starting dose was always 4 capsules per day, each containing either 25 mg aprindine or placebo. But the dose could be adjusted upwards to a maximum of 8 capsules/day, the primary reason to do so being persistence of arrhythmias, or downwards to 2 capsules/day, suspected side effects being the reason. Decisions to adjust were taken by the principal investigators without breaking the double-blinding. Apart from a base-line 24-hour ECG to establish eligibility, 24-hour ECGs were repeated after 1, 3 and 6 months and at the conclusion of follow-up, i.e. at 12 months.

The results of the GRAP-study may be regarded as typical for this type of arrhythmia trial. At base-line, the two treatment groups were well balanced with reference to age, sex, size and location of infarct (as evidenced by enzyme levels) and clinical course during hospitalization. In a considerable proportion of patients in both groups, treatment was discontinued prematurely because of suspected toxicity or refusal of the patient (29/151 in the aprindine group, 18/149 in the placebo group). In terms of persistence of arrhythmias, there were marked differences between the groups. In the aprindine group, the percentage of patients who still had complex ventricular arrhythmias ranged from 47% to 51%, depending on the time of 24-hour ECG follow-up. In the placebo group, the same percentage ranged from 75% − 83% ($p < 0.001$, Mantel-Haenszel chi-square test with one degree of freedom). These results reflect both the already known anti-arrhythmic effect of aprindine and the "spontaneous" disappearance of arrhythmias when patients are selected on the basis of their presence ("regression-to-the-mean").

Notwithstanding the difference in terms of arrhythmias, there was no statistically significant difference in terms of the primary endpoint. While still treated, the number of cardiac sudden deaths (defined in this case as death within 24 hours without apparent non-cardiac cause) or episodes of documented VF was 10 in the aprindine group and 12 in the placebo group.

Corresponding total number of deaths were 10 and 17, which difference again was not statistically significant.

A "Negative" Study: What Does It Mean?

Today, not many people will still make the mistake of believing that a "non-significant difference" proves that there is in fact no difference between the treatments which are compared. One obvious alternative explanation is almost invariably that a so-called type II or β error may have been made or, in other words, that the size of the study was too small to have a reasonable chance to detect a difference if in fact one existed. In that case, "negative" is really a mis-nomer, "non-informative" being the more appropriate adjective. For the results of the GRAP-study discussed above, a type II error is a perfectly reasonable explanation, especially since the SD-rate actually observed was much lower than the one on which sample size calculations were based (a not uncommon feature of clinical trials . . .). The question is whether there are other explanations for a negative anti-arrhythmic trial.

We would probably not have considered this problem, had it not been for one particular observation made while analyzing the data from the GRAP-study. In this study, 24-hour ECGs were repeated after 1, 3, 6 and 12 months. Therefore, for patients who died suddenly or had documented VF after the first month of follow-up, a 24-hour ECG was available which preceded the event. It appeared that of 14 such events, all but one were preceded by a 24-hour ECG which still showed the presence of complex ventricular arrhythmias. This observation suggests that the disappearance of complex ventricular arrhythmias, whether "spontaneous" or as a result of aprindine treatment, carries an excellent prognosis. From the results of the GRAP-study therefore, we were left with what seems a paradox: a with respect to suppression of arrhythmias effective treatment (though not always so), an excellent prognosis when the complex arrhythmias which were present at the start of treatment disappear, but no end-point difference in the only valid comparison which can be made, i.e. the one between the aprindine and placebo groups.

Taking patients with complex arrhythmias as starting point, the paradox referred to above can, apart by a type II error, readily be explained also if one assumes that the treatment results in (i) a lowered SD-rate in patients who have their arrhythmias suppressed, and (ii) a raised SD-rate due to some toxic effect in patients in whom the arrhythmias persist despite treatment. If one accepts this explanation as a reasonable hypothesis, the conclusion must be that anti-arrhythmic trials such as the GRAP-study will, by virtue of their design, never give the answer. The reason for this may need some explanation. To verify the above hypothesis, or falsify it, it is necessary to determine the effect of anti-arrhythmic treatment on the SD-rate *conditional on* the effect of the drug on the arrhythmia. To put it differently, one needs to show that the SD-rate is decreased in patients who have their arrhythmia successfully controlled and is not affected, or even increased, in patients in whom this is not the case. This can be done only if the results of a secondary preventive trial like the GRAP-study can be stratified by what may be called the intermediary treatment effect, in this case the effect on the arrhythmias. It probably needs not much further explanation that the design of the GRAP-study, and of similar studies, does not allow for such stratification if it is remembered that the anti-arrhythmic effect on the treatment becomes apparent only after randomization has taken place. Stratification is possible only for variables which are known at the moment of randomization. For the variable "suppression of arrhythmia", this is never the case in the type of study considered here.

An Alternative Study Design: A Proposal

A study design which would overcome the problems alluded to above, would involve the following steps:
1. Selection of patients on the basis of presence of CHD and arrhythmias, as documented by for instance a 24-hour ECG
2. A period of open treatment with the chosen study drug, during which the dosis can be titrated and patients with apparent side-effects are excluded
3. Assessment of the apparent effect on the arrhythmias detected at step 1 by a repeat 24-hour ECG
4. Randomization to either continuation on active treatment at the dose achieved during step 2 or to placebo.

A few comments to this only in general terms outlined design are made here. Obviously, only a drug with proven anti-arrhythmic properties should be used. Ideally, those properties should be documented in the frame work of a short-term randomized study of sufficient sample size to reasonably exclude the possibility that the period of open treatment is in fact a mortality risk to the patient. At step 4, one has the choice to randomize only those patients in whom suppression of arrhythmia may be assumed on the basis of an intrapatient comparison of the 24-hour ECGs made at step 1 and 3. Alternatively, all patients could be randomized so that the effect on mortality can be studied also for those patients who did not react to the treatment in terms of the intermediary treatment effect, i.e. disappearance of arrhythmias. Also, the possibility exists to repeat step 2 with a different drug in the "non-responders" at step 3, again going to step 4 only if this choice proves to suppress the arrhythmia. Particular attention will have to be paid then to the definition of "non-responders". In this context an important consideration will be the natural variability of arrhythmias, as discussed by Dr. Prineas. (4)

Conclusions

In our opinion, studies as outlined above should be done. They are the only basis on which the present argument pro and contra anti-arrhythmic treatment in the prevention of SD can be settled. One of the reasons is that only such a study puts current clinical practice with anti-arrhythmic drugs, in which the intermediary treatment effect on the arrhythmia itself plays an important role, to a real test. A final argument mentioned here is that only such a study will contribute to our knowledge about the mechanism of VF and the role of PVCs in that mechanism.

The concept of a "running-in-period" in clinical trials, as used in the proposed study, is by no means a new one. The need to incorporate such a period deserves however renewed attention.

References

1. Lown B: Sudden Cardiac Death: The Major Challenge Confronting Contemporary Cardiology. Am Jrn Cardiology 43: 313–328, 1979.
2. Hagemeijer F, Glaser B, Van Durme JP, Bogaert M: Design of a Study to Evaluate Drug Therapy of Serious Ventricular Rhythm Disturbances After an Acute Myocardial Infarction. Europ J Cardiol 6: 299–310, 1977.
3. Prineas RJ: this publication.

TESTING THE EFFICACY OF ANTIARRHYTHMIC THERAPY

R.J. PRINEAS

Introduction

We have already heard in this symposium of the success to date of recent anti-arrhythmia trials (1), and of the most likely groups of patients in which to test the efficacy of antiarrhythmic drugs (2). Other problems of design have been presented earlier (3). This presentation is concerned with requirements for judging the effect of such therapy in controlled clinical trials for people at high risk of sudden death after an acute myocardial infarction.

Although the effectiveness of long-term therapy in post-myocardial infarction (MI) patients is only acceptable if an improvement in mortality can be demonstrated (3, 4) measurement of the presence of arrhythmias is an important intermediate endpoint that must be addressed in all such trials. This presentation is restricted to the discussion of such measurement. In some past randomized controlled trials of antiarrhythmic drugs in post-MI patients, that monitored arrhythmias, the drugs decreased the incidence of ventricular arrhythmias and ventricular premature beats (VPB) without significantly changing mortality (5, 6). Dr. Lubsen has developed this theme (2). Why then is monitoring of arrhythmias needed in a randomized controlled clinical trial of antiarrhythmic agents? There are at least four reasons:

1) identifying risk subgroups
2) safety
3) elucidating mechanisms
4) natural history studies

1. Identifying Risk Sub-groups

Among post-MI patients there are groups with ventricular arrhythmias, found on monitoring prior to hospital discharge, that have a substantially increased risk of sudden death. It is in these groups that antiarrhythmic therapy preventing the onset of ventricular fibrillation (VF) "should be" most effective. Future trials might concentrate first on this group or at least use stratified randomization with a large enough sample size to detect an effect in this group.

How should the arrhythmias be identified prior to hospital discharge? Frequent VPB preceding VF is the most common ventricular arrhythmic finding in the coronary care unit (CCU) (7, 8). This subject has recently been extensively reviewed by Moss (9). He and others (34) have concluded that in the early stages of myocardial infarction there are no clear warning arrhythmias based on VPB morphology or timing that identify patients at high risk of VF in the CCU. Again, the likelihood of further inhospital VF after discharge from the CCU is associated more with the state of the myocardium – the size and location of the infarct, left ventricular function and heart failure. However, Holter monitoring in the post-hospital and predischarge period has identified high risk groups for sudden death based on independent prediction of specific ventricular arrhythmias.

1.1. Holter Monitoring

Holter monitoring has been carried out in the post-hospital phase of myocardial infarction and the prognosis of various ventricular arrhythmias determined in this way has also recently been reviewed by Moss (9). The results of all of these studies showed a two to threefold increase in risk associated with complex VPB for future cardiac death over one to three years of follow-up. More recently Ruberman, et al (10) have shown that five year mortality from sudden cardiac death in 1,739 post-MI men is independently related to complex VPB found on baseline Holter monitoring within nine months of the entry infarct. They found that men with R-on-T or runs of two or more VPB in the hour had a more than fourfold increase (25% vs 6%) in sudden coronary death (within minutes) compared to men free of any VPB in the hour. Additionally, complex VPB, R-on-T, runs of two or more, multiform or bigeminy carried a more than twofold risk of non sudden coronary mortality in the ensuing five years. Although those with complex VPB formed only 27% of the men they accounted for about half the number of sudden deaths. Moss and colleagues (9, 11) have proposed a refinement of Ruberman's grading system based on 940 patients with acute myocardial infarction who had six hour Holter monitoring before discharge from hospital. Independent contributions to predicting total mortality suggested a grading system of:

Low risk: 1) No VPB
2) Uniform VPB with late-cycle (R-R$'$/QT > 1.0)
High risk VPB: 3) Uniform VPB with early-cycle (R-R$'$/QT $\leqslant 1.0$)
4) Multiform VPB

They found that if multiformity or early-cycle VPB were present frequency did not add to the prediction. When multiform or early-cycle VPB were controlled for, frequency, bigeminal patterns or repetitive VPB were not found to have independent prognostic value. The grading was based on total mortality and not sudden death. A comparison with the modified Lown (12) grading system and the Ruberman (10) grading system showed a greater discrimination for Moss's high and low risk groups. The high risk VPB were independent of age, education, social class, history of cigarette smoking, history of angina, history of myocardial infarction, NYHA Classification II, III, IV, site of infarct or left ventricular dysfunction.

Of these predictive factors, those independent of high risk VPB were: NYHA Classification II III IV, history of angina, history of myocardial infarction, anterior site for the acute infarction and left ventricular dysfunction. This is not dissimilar to the findings of Ruberman, et al, (10) who found the most important predictors for future sudden death (controlling for complex VPB) were: congestive failure, ST-T depression and heart rate.

Neither Ruberman nor Moss examined the independent prognosis of prolonged QT intervals. Earlier studies of Lown, et al (13), and Han and Goel (14) suggested prematurity indices that are more ominous with prolonged QT intervals. And more recently Schwartz and Wolfs (15) showed that prolonged QT intervals were associated with a greater risk of sudden death. However, this study was confounded by the use of antiarrhythmic drugs.

Differences in Moss and Ruberman's finding might relate to different times since entry MI, different length of monitoring or different definitions of sudden death. Bigger, et al (16) also discuss the inadequacy of the Lown (12) classification to identify those at risk. Their suggestion is: "In the present state of knowledge it seems more reasonable to assess the risk of various (VPB) characteristics separately and then to combine these variables and frequency with other characteristics of ischemic heart disease in the search for a combination which best identifies those at highest risk to subsequent sudden death." Until more analyses or results of observational studies are available high risk groups may be chosen from patients with early cycle VPB or multiform VPB.

1.2. Duration of Monitoring

How long a monitoring period should be used? Moss (9) used six hours and Ruberman (10) only one hour. Some have pleaded for very much longer periods of monitoring. Morganroth and colleagues in a series of papers (19–21) have well demonstrated the variability of ventricular ectopy hour-to-hour and day-to-day in patients with cardiac disease. Others (17, 18) have also found similar variability. Preselection of 15 patients with various cardiac disorders with VPB $\geq$ 30/hours over 24 hours, monitored on three successive days off antiarrhythmic drugs (19) enabled patients to be ranked by VPB frequency because the major source of variations was "between patients". Over a three day period nearly half of the variability from day-to-day was due to the hour-to-hour variability. Using this data the authors projected that a minimal change in frequency to detect a significant change in VPB frequency for 24 hour monitoring required an 83.4% reduction when compared with one "test" 24 hour monitoring period. This was under controlled clinic conditions in clinically stable patients. They also noted, however, that the higher the rate of VPB occurrence the less the variability. In a further study to elicit the variability of complex VPB, this same group (20) made four consecutive 24 hour recordings in 20 patients. Again, these patients were preselected and had an earlier 24 hour recording with ⩾ 30 VPB/hour. The patients had differing cardiac diseases, were clinically stable and were monitored as outpatients. The authors examined the variability of couplets and runs of three or more VPB, but not of "R-on-T" or multiform VPB. Variability was examined for each eight hour period for each of the four days. Like VPB frequency the greatest variability was "between patients" and for individual patients "between hours" rather than "between days" or "between 8-hour periods". From this data they projected a minimum percentage decrease in complex VPB or ventricular tachycardia to be achieved by antiarrhythmic therapy for a significant change to be a 75% reduction for couplets and a 65% reduction for ventricular tachycardia using one control 24 hour monitoring and one test 24 hour monitoring. The study also showed a statistically significant reduction in the frequency of couplets or ventricular tachycardia during sleep compared to the rest of the day. The authors argue that the variability of these complex ventricular arrhythmias in individual patients is so great that "it may be inadvisable to pool data to detect trends in ectopic frequency in evaluating new potential antiarrhythmic agents in groups of patients."

In a later article Morganroth extends this argument (21) and gives recommended guidelines to test therapeutic efficacy of antiarrhythmic drugs in individual patients. He recommends repeat ambulatory monitoring "only after the patient has received an adequate dose of an antiarrhythmic agent and has reached a steady state." He further recommends that repeat monitoring must be carried out to be certain that the drug continues to be efficacious and that "periodic discontinuation" of the drug with repeated Holter monitoring be used to determine whether or not ventricular dysarrhythmias continue to be present! Morganroth's studies do not examine longer term variability and they were not done in post-MI patients. Further, the dangers referred to are only those outside statistical control achievable in randomized trials.

Ruberman, et al (22) in a further analysis of their data in 1,445 men in the first nine months after acute myocardial infarction with repeat one hour monitoring on repeat occasions, six months apart, showed a constant − 25% − proportion of men on each occasion had complex ventricular rhythm (R-on-T, bigeminy, multiform, runs of two or more VPB) and that approximately 50% had such rhythms on both occasions whereas only 15% had complex rhythms on the second occasion but not the first.

Winkle and colleagues (23) have recently reported results of three consecutive 24 hour Holter monitoring in 57 patients 8–11 days post-MI. On any given recording day for the group there was approximately the same prevalence of each type of complex arrhythmia (day 1: multiform 49%, R-on-T 32%, pairs 18%, bigeminy 25%, ventricular tachycardia (VT) 11%, and any complex VPB 67%).

Within-hour accumulation of patients with complex ventricular rhythms showed that by 24 hours 86% of patients with any VPB had been detected. The additional yield from 48 to 72 hours was greatest for VT detection — 42% of such patients were detected only during the final 24 hour recording. The frequency of VPB per hour in each of the 3x24 hour recording was most reproducible for high rates of VPB so that only 67% of those with rates below two per hour were at this level on all three days. Whereas, of those with rates at or above five per hour 86% to 90% were at these rates on all three days. For complex VPB those showing a particular type of complex rhythm on all three days varied from 63% for multiform or any complex VPB to 81% of those with VT. They pointed out that because Ruberman's data on prognostic significance is based on one hour of monitoring and that those patients with complex VPB in a shorter duration of monitoring are likely to have a higher frequency of these rhythms on further monitoring it may be that those with the most frequent complex rhythms are at highest risk of subsequent sudden death. There is not sufficient published data to clarify this.

Both Ruberman and Moss showed that complex forms were more likely with increasing VPB frequency. However, in Winkle's population all patients with VPB greater than 100 in 24 hours had complex VPB. Conversely they found that 65% of patients with only two to ten VPB in a 24 hour recording also had complex forms present.

If frequency of complex forms rather than just presence or absence is the most important predictive factor for sudden death in post-MI patients then a shorter duration (than 72 hours) will be adequate to identify an at risk group. Earlier studies clearly show an increased prevalence of ventricular arrhythmias with increased monitoring periods (24).

Thanavaro, et al (25) in a small group of patients showed that the presence of frequent or complex VPB is directly related to the logarithm of the recording duration and a 12-hour recording will uncover 95% of those with frequent VPB in any hour of 24 hours and 84% of multiform VPB. These results are notably different from Winkle's.

1.3. Other Recording Methods

There are other methods of uncovering high risk arrhythmias than Holter monitoring. Use of stress testing in post infarct survivors to examine the predictive value of arrhythmias uncovered during exercise has been recently extensively reviewed (9, 24, 26). Like Holter monitoring, stress testing is noninvasive and though it carries some risk has been more and more used in post-MI patients. It is the summary of each of these reviews that 24 hour ambulatory monitoring uncovers more ventricular arrhythmias than exercise testing in both the early and late post infarct period. There is overlap with ambulatory monitoring, and exercise-induced arrhythmias have independent value for predicting mortality (42). Both methods together uncover more patients with VPB than either method alone.

And one study (27) showed isometric exercise uncovered more arrhythmias than dynamic exercise.

ST segment depression uncovered by treadmill testing, at the time of hospital discharge post-MI, has demonstrated a 16-fold increased risk of sudden death in one year after myocardial infarction (28). Prognostic information of ST segment depression measured from Holter recordings has not been obtained. Therefore, exercise testing and ambulatory monitoring are complementary procedures for detecting post-MI patients at risk of sudden death.

Detecting high risk myocardial states for malignant ventricular arrhythmias may in the future require far more detailed measurement than Holter recording analysis. Acute MI patients that have a repetitive ventricular response to stimulation via a temporary transvenous pacemaker have a particularly high rate of sudden death in the following twelve months (29–31). However, this is a risky procedure that would require an enormous effort in a large clinical trial with varying capabilities to apply it safely in multiple centers. Such methods as body surface mapping of QRST area (32) are also unlikely for the present to be logistically possible in large clinical trials.

2. Safety

Monitoring of arrhythmias in clinical trials is as important for detecting unwanted side effects of "antiarrhythmic" drugs as for testing their efficacy. Some antiarrhythmic drugs may actually increase the frequency or occurrence of some arrhythmias (33). In order to test the arrhythmogenic effect of these agents there should be a monitoring period at the end of a trial after study medication has been stopped.

3. Elucidating Mechanisms

It an antiarrhythmic agent is shown by a trial to prevent sudden death, without repeat monitoring for arrhythmias during the course of one trial it would be impossible to judge if the outcome depended on the ability of the agent to suppress certain ventricular arrhythmias. The question is how often and for what period should monitoring be repeated?

Ruberman and colleagues (22) have shown the relative stability of complex VPB when repeating one hour monitoring at six month intervals in post-MI patients. However, the baseline monitoring in their studies started only after discharge from hospital and up to nine months post infarction. Nevertheless, comparison of their finding of "complex arrhythmias" at baseline and Moss's (9) "high risk" arrhythmias in the predischarge, six-hour monitoring periods are similar enough to suppose for the moment that predischarge arrhythmias are likely to be relatively stable without therapy during the first year out of hospital for myocardial infarction survivors.

The first monitoring after the baseline period should probably occur early for reasons of safety. Also, given that sudden death rates are highest in the first six months after discharge the first repeat monitoring should occur early in this period. A case can also be made for repeat monitoring within one month of baseline to adjust the dosage of an antiarrhythmic drug rather than using only blood levels to establish an optimal dose for the remainder of the trial. The duration of monitoring should probably be the same as that used at baseline.

Very large numbers of patients, treated in multiple centers, usually need to be recruited when mortality is used as the primary endpoint in post-MI trials. This puts cost and measurement error limitations on the length of time for monitoring both at baseline and subsequently. The data on prevalence and stability of ventricular arrhythmias in post-MI patients comes from dedicated research centers where measurement variability is kept to a minimum. The more quantitative the desired analysis of ventricular arrhythmias the more crucial is quality control (35). Also, repeatability for detecting qualitative descriptors, R-on-T and multiform is relatively poor (35). These problems would argue for longer rather than shorter periods of monitoring. However, variability of ventricular arrhythmia occurrence is also affected by eating, physical activity, drugs and psychological state. All of these must be recorded in a diary during the monitoring period, if it is long, and so adds to the complexity of the analysis.

We may also need more and more factorial design for post-MI trials in the future (36), i.e., testing multiple drugs in the one trial. We have particular warning for this in a recent study from Norway (37), where Timolol (a noncardioselective beta-blocking agent) was administered to post-MI patients in a randomized, double-blind trial. The incidence of both sudden death and reinfarction was significantly reduced. Treatment was started 7–28 days after infarction in 945 patients on Timolol and 939 patients on placebo and patients were followed for 12 to 33 months. However, warnings not to act on the result of this one trial until the results of several other post-myocardial infarction studies are available have already been sounded (38, 39). Nevertheless, the study includes the real possibility of future controlled trials taking place without a placebo group. In such situations, monitoring periods would have to be extended considerably to detect significant differences in arrhythmia occurrence between new and "established" therapies. It might be that in such a case the hope of detecting significant differences in arrhythmias or change in arrhythmias, will be impossible with 24-hour monitoring.

Recording of changes in high risk ventricular rhythms can be done by examining changes in the proportions of patients in each treatment group who have these arrhythmias. However, because the importance of the frequency of these abnormalities is not yet settled then some index of frequency should also be compared between the groups. The question of whether suppression of frequent VPB also suppresses complex forms can also be tested. The comparison of mean frequencies for any VPB or high risk VPB between groups might be confounded by a few patients with very high frequencies in either group. This can be overcome by a ranking of frequency of any arrhythmia of interest and using non-parametric statistics or a two-sample t-test with a transformation of the new ranked frequency variable (x) to log (x+1) for arrhythmias that are absent from many patients, such as might occur with some of the high risk VPB. The range of frequencies to be compared at each level can be determined by examining the distribution of VPB frequency at baseline. Quantitative measures of prematurity such as $R\text{-}R_i/QT > 1.0$ are prefarable to qualitative descriptions such as "R-on-T". The repeatability is likely to be higher for the former.

Frequencies can be counted per monitoring period. However, both Moe and colleagues (40) and Hinkle (41) make a plea for recording VPB frequency in relation to the frequency of all beats rather than as a rate expressed over time. This is because a ventricular arrhythmia may be apparently abolished with a change in heart rate without any direct effect on the abnormal mechanism; the frequency of the VPB may change with changing heart rate and so confound comparisons of rates per time; and finally, because some analysis programs eliminate periods of artifact so that the number of VPB counted in a given time period may be falsely high.

4. Natural History Studies

The "definitive trial" for any therapy is generally an impossible goal. So that each clinical trial should suggest ways of improving therapy by targeting more precisely on high risk subgroups. In the course of this presentation it has been pointed out that there are still unanswered questions about the risk of QT interval length, frequency of *any* VPB, *frequency* of early-cycle or multiform VPB, ST segment depression measured from Holter recordings and arrhythmias occurring during sleep. By finding answers to these questions we can better define high risk groups for future clinical trials and for the clinical setting. The cost and time of mounting natural history studies in isolation, to answer these questions, inhibits rapid progress. For this reason, in all large scale clinical trials, efforts should be encouraged to collect data that will increase our knowledge in these areas.

Conclusion

From the foregoing it seems reasonable to suggest for the immediate future trials, baseline Holter monitorings of 24 hours with repeat 24 hour monitorings at three months and annually for the duration of the trial. In addition, a repeat 24 hour monitoring one month after study medication has been stopped could be done to determine adverse arrhythmogenic effects attributable to the study medications. Statistical calculations to estimate the sample size needed to detect expected changes in frequency should be made in an effort to reduce the logistics and cost problems associated with such large scale monitoring efforts. It may be that after baseline only a subsample of the participants needs to be monitored.

No one has yet addressed the problem of combining exercise tests with Holter monitoring in an antiarrhythmic trial. To do so requires consideration of a balance of yield, cost, standardization of the exercise test in multiple centers and risk of the procedure itself though exercise tests have been demonstrated to be well tolerated.

References

1. Van Durme JP, 1981. Clinical evaluation of therapeutic interventions to prevent premature cardiac death. This symposium.
2. Lubsen J, 1981. Design of clinical trials related to Holter electrocardiography. This symposium.
3. Prineas RJ, 1975. Problems in Design and Evaluation of Antiarrhythmia Trials. Circulation Suppl 3 to *51* & *52*, 248.
4. May GS, Eberlein KA, Furberg CD, Passamani ER, DeMets DL, 1981. Secondary Prevention After Myocardial Infarction: A review of Long-Term Trials, in press, Progress in Cardiovascular Diseases.
5. Collaborative Group, 1971: Phenytoin after recovery from myocardial infarction: Controlled trial in 568 patients. Lancet *2*: 1055.
6. Peter T, Ross D, Duffield A, Luxton M, Harper R, Hunt D, Sloman G, 1978. Effect on survival after myocardial infarction of longterm treatment with phenytoin. Br Heart J *40*: 1356.
7. Lown B, Fakhro AM, Hood WB Jr., Thorn GW, 1967. The coronary care unit. New Perspectives and directions. JAMA 199: 188.
8. Lown, B, Kosowsky BD, Klein MD, 1969. Pathogenesis, prevention, and treatment of arrhythmias in myocardial infarction. Circulation 39 and 40 (Suppl) 4: 261.
9. Moss AJ, 1980. Clinical significance of ventricular arrhythmias in patients with or without coronary artery disease. Progress in Cardiovascular Diseases *23*: 33.
10. Ruberman W, Weinblatt E, Goldberg JD, Frank CW, Chardhary BS, Shapiro S. 1981. Ventricular premature complexes and sudden death after myocardial infarction. Circulation *64*: 297.
11. Davis HT, Moss AJ, De Camilla JJ, 1981. Ambulatory ECG recording: Prognostic value. In: *Ambulatory Electrocardiographic Recording*, Wenger NK, Mock MB and Ringquist I, Year Book Medical Publishers Inc. (Chicago), pp. 391.
12. Lown B, Wolf M, 1971. Approaches to sudden death from coronary heart disease. Circulation *44*: 130.
13. Lown B, Klein MD, Hershberg PI, 1969. Coronary and precoronary care. Am J Med *46*: 705.
14. Han J, Goel BG, 1972. Electrophysiologic precursors of ventricular tachyarrhythmias. Arch Int Med *129*: 749.
15. Schwartz PJ, Wolfs, 1978. QT interval prolongation as a predictor of sudden death in patients with myocardial infarction. Circulation *57*: 1074.
16. Bigger JR, Wenger TL, Heissenbuttel RHJ, 1977. Limitations of the Lown grading system for the study of human ventricular arrhythmias. Am Heart J *93*: 727.
17. Misner JE, Inrey PB, Smith L, et al. 1978. Secular variation in frequency of premature ventricular contractions in untreated individuals. J Lab Clin Med 92: 117.
18. Engler R, Ryan W, LeWinter, et al, 1974. Assessment of long-term antiarrhythmic therapy. Studies on the long-term efficacy and toxicity of tocainide. Am J Cardiol 43: 612.

19. Morganroth J, 1981. Optimal use of long-term ambulatory electrocardiographic monitoring. Cardiovascular Revs and Reps *2*: 333.
20. Michelson EL, Morganroth J, 1980. Spontaneous variability of complex ventricular arrhythmias detected by long-term electrocardiographic recording. Circulation *61*: 690.
21. Morganroth JL, Michelson, Horowitz LN, Josephson MD, Pearlman AS, Dunkman WB, 1978. Limitations of routine long-term electrocardiographic monitoring to assess ventricular ectopic frequency. Circulation 58: 408.
22. Ruberman W, Weinblatt E, Frank CW, Goldberg JD, Shapiro S, 1981. Repeated 1-hour electrocardiographic monitoring of survivors of myocardial infarction at six month intervals: arrhythmia detection and relation to prognosis. The Amer J Cardiol *47*: 1197.
23. Winkle RA, Peters F, Hall R, 1981. Characterization of ventricular tachyarrhythmias on ambulatory ECG recordings in post-myocardial infarction patients: Arrhythmia detection and duration of recording relationship between arrhythmia frequency and complexity, and day-to-day reproducibility. Amer Heart J *102*: 162.
24. Kennedy HL, 1981. Comparison of ambulatory electrocardiography and exercise testing. The Amer J Cardiol *47*: 1359.
25. Thanavaro S, Kleiger RE, Hieb BR, Krone RJ, deMollo VR, Oliver C, 1980. Effect of electrocardiographic recording duration on ventricular dysrhythmia detection after myocardial infarction. Circulation *62*: 262.
26. Winkle RA, 1981. Ventricular arrhythmias: Clinical aspects. In: *Ambulatory Electrocardiographic Recording*, Wenger NK, Mock MB and Ringquist I, Years Book Medical Publishers Inc. (Chicago), pp. 259.
27. Atkins JM, Matthews OA, Blomqvist CG, Mullins CB, 1976. Incidence of arrhythmias induced by isometric and dynamic exercise. Br Heart J *38*: 465.
28. Theroux P, Waters DD, Halphen C, Debaisieux JC, Mizgala HF, 1979. Prognostic value of exercise testing soon after myocardial infarction N Engl J Med *301*: 341.
29. Kastor JA, Horowitz LN, Harken AH, Josephson ME, 1981. Clinical Electrophysiology of ventricular tachycardia. N Eng J Med *304*: 1004.
30. Greene HL, Reid PR, Shaeffer AH, 1978. The repetitive ventricular response in man. A prediction of sudden death. N Engl J Med *299*: 729.
31. Ruskin JN, DiMarco JP, Garan H, 1980. Out-of-hospital cardiac arrest: Electrophysiologic observations and selection of long-term antiarrhythmic therapy. N Engl J Med *303*: 607.
32. Abildskov JA, 1980. Recognition of cardiac states at high risk of ventricular arrhythmias by means of electrocardiographic wave form. Japanese Circulation Journal *44*: 691.
33. Montgomery BJ, 1979. Antiarrhythmic agents may cause sudden death: Drug testing urged. JAMA *245*: 1771.
34. Campbell R, Murray A, Julian DG, 1978. Incidence, prevalence and significance of ventricular ectopic activity in acute myocardial infarction in Sande E, Julian DG, Bell JW (eds): Management of Ventricular Tachycardia – Role of Mexiletine. Amsterdam, Exerpta Medica, pp. 457.
35. Crow RS, Prineas RJ, 1981. Quality control. In: *Ambulatory Electrocardiographic Recording*, Wenger NK, Mock MB and Ringquist I, Year Book Medical Publishers Inc. (Chicago), pp. 391.
36. Armitage P, 1980. Clinical trials in the secondary prevention of myocardial infarction and stroke. Thrombosis and Haemostasis *43*: 90.
37. The Norwegian Multicenter Study Group, 1981. Timolol-induced reduction in mortality and reinfarction in patients surviving myocardial infarction. N Eng J Med *304*: 801.
38. Braunwald E, 1981. Comments. Intelligence Reports in Cardiovascular Disease July issue, pp. 5.
39. Lancet, 1981. Beta-blockers after myocardial infarction. *1*: 873.
40. Moe GK, Jalife J, Antzelevitch F, 1981. Ventricular arrhythmias: Evaluation of mechanisms. In: *Ambulatory Electrocardiographic Recording*, Wenger NK, Mock MB and Ring-

quist I, Year Book Medical Publishers Inc. (Chicago), pp. 243.

41. Hinkle LE, 1981. Arrhythmia evaluation: Commentary. In: *Ambulatory Electrocardiographic Recording*, Wenger NK, Mock MB and Ringquist I, Year Book MedicalPublishers Inc. (Chicago), pp. 299.

42. Weld FM, Chu K, Bigger JT, Rolnitzky LM, 1981. Risk stratification with low-level exercise testing two weeks after acute myocardial infarction. Circulation *64*: 306.

TRANSLATING RESULTS OF CLINICAL TRIALS INTO CLINICAL RELEVANCE

DESMOND G. JULIAN

Both statisticians and drug companies are often surprised and, perhaps, disappoint-ed to find that clinicians do not always translate the apparently clear-cut results of clinical trials into their daily practice. In this presentation, I will endeavour to examine why it is that physicians, in general, and cardiologists in particular, are, and indeed should be, hesitant about extrapolating from published trials into real life.

The conduct of clinical trials has developed into a major industry and numerous experts throughout the world have written clear and detailed instructions on how to design and analyse them. As I am not one of them, I am not going to endeavour to tackle this aspect of the problem at length, but one must say that there are many trials still being published which do not fulfill the accepted require-ments. These will be discussed, but attention will be directed at aspects that have been neglected because they are seldom considered by statisticians and epi-demiologists.

Design and Analysis Faults

One of the major reasons for not accepting the conclusions reached by trialists is doubt about their scientific merit.

Undoubtedly, the biggest fault in trials which have been undertaken in recent years is that of insufficient sample size (1, 2). This has led to the widespread conclusion that certain trials, such as those on beta-blockers have been "negative", when such a deduction cannot legitimately be made. This kind of error has led to such conclusions as "anticoagulants are no use after myocardial infarction", "the propranolol study after myocardial infarction was negative" and "the anti-hypertensive trials have shown that the control of hypertension does not lead to a fall in the incidence of coronary disease".

Of course, another reason why trials, which on their face value are impressive, have failed to lead to changes in clinical practice is when a trial is considered not to be valid. The most recent famous example of this is the Anturane Reinfarction

Trial (3); grave doubts have been cast on the correctness of the analysis and it is now fairly clear that Anturane did not lead to a significant reduction in death in this trial — either sudden or secondary to myocardial infarction.

Another factor which leads to doubts about the relevance of a trial relates to the definition of the population being studied. This is a problem that is now being widely recognised but it is unfortunate that in the past so many studies have been undertaken which do not allow us to know what segment of the whole population at risk was selected. These observations apply to the Multicentre International Trial of practolol (4) and the European Coronary Artery Bypass Trial (5).

The Creation of a Problem that did not exist before

Another reason for the non-acceptance of trials is that they may be dealing with a problem that is clinically non-existent. In this context, it is worth considering the ventricular ectopic beat as a cause of symptoms. We all know from material presented at this and other meetings, that ventricular ectopic rhythms are extremely common in the normal population and even more so in the middle-aged elderly coronary population. The vast majority of these episodes are entirely asymptomatic and although ventricular arrhythmias are one of the commonest manifestations of coronary disease, palpitation and syncope are two of its rarest symptomatic presentations. Is it not astonishing that virtually all patients have ventricular arrhythmias and about 50 per cent have serious ventricular arrhythmias in the first 48 hours of myocardial infarction, but complaints because of these arrhythmias are exceedingly rare! In our experience, it is also rare for patients to complain of symptoms which can be directly related to ventricular arrhythmias during the convalescent phase of infarction unless their attention has been drawn to the possibility. Undoubtedly, Holter monitoring has led to an upsurge in complaints of patients for once attention is drawn to the possibility of palpitation, it is commonly complained of. We have an ironic situation, therefore, with Holter monitoring being responsible for the provocation of symptoms which then require the use of otherwise unnecessary antiarrhythmic drugs, whose effectiveness then has to be evaluated by further Holter monitoring.

The Relevance of End-points studied to the Clinical Problem

In many cases, it is not easy to study the clinical problem directly. Other end-points are, therefore, chosen which are assumed to relate to it. A most conspicuous example of this is the relationship of ventricular arrhythmias to death and, particularly, sudden death. A very large part of the Holter monitoring industry has developed on the assumption that ventricular arrhythmias are important as causes of death. This matter is far from resolved. There is no doubt of course that the ability to show on Holter monitoring the suppression of episodes of recurrent sustained ventricular tachycardia or fibrillation is relevant to the prevention of such episodes in the future. But these cases are rare. Much more important are the high-risk patients after infarction with ventricular arrhythmias often associated with left ventricular dysfunction; it is far from clear what the relationship is between such ventricular arrhythmias and sudden death. Thus in the mexiletine trial (6) which we undertook, there was a clear-cut reduction in ventricular ectopic activity but no reduction in death, although it must be admitted that the size of the trial was too small to make a categorical deduction about this. What is of considerable interest in this context is that some of the newer antiarrhythmic drugs, such as encainide (7) and flecainide (8), are outstandingly successful in achieving total suppression of ventricular ectopic activity but there is evidence to suggest that they are more likely to aggravate ventricular tachycardias than, for example, less "effective" drugs such as mexiletine and tocainide. On the other hand, the two forms of therapy which appear to be most effective in preventing sudden death – timolol (9) and coronary artery bypass surgery (5) – are therapies which have little or no effect on ventricular arrhythmias as detected by Holter monitoring.

One can foresee a further problem in this regard in the near future with regard to the effect of drug therapy on asymptomatic ST changes. There is certainly evidence that these asymptomatic ST changes are often if not always associated with myocardial ischaemia, but what the relevance of drug treatment in suppressing these changes is to the control of myocardial ischaemia and its long-term effects will be difficult to assess.

Quality and Control of Therapy in the Trial compared with Clinical Practice

Patients in clinical trials are not treated in the same way as they would be if they were being treated by their own physician in daily practice. There are numerous ways in which this can be illustrated.

Perhaps the most obvious is the selection of a particular dosage of a drug for an individual patient. There are few trials which can make allowances for individual variations in response to therapy and even where such attempts have been made, it is assumed that once an "effective" dose for that patients is achieved this will remain stable whereas variations in dosage of such drugs as digoxin, diuretics and nitrates are frequently required.

This problem is particularly relevant when two forms of active therapy are being compared. I certainly know of one study comparing calcium blockers with beta-blockers in which the calcium blocker dosage is probably optimal whereas the beta-blockers dosage is sub-optimal. In such circumstances, the trial is slanted adversely in relation to the beta-blocker.

Another problem in trials is the question of quality control. In the case of surgical trials, it is relatively easy to see whether standards of therapy are what could or should be expected. However, it was apparent in the Veterans Administration trial of coronary artery surgery (10), that the mortality was substantially higher than even moderately good clinics at that time would accept and this seriously vitiated the deductions from that trial. Even in the European Coronary Artery Bypass trial (5), with a mortality in good risk cases of something over 3 per cent, questions were raised about the quality of the surgery. Indeed, in the latter part of the trial the surgical mortality fell to 1.5 per cent. On the other hand, it is wrong to extrapolate to general use the results from the outstandingly good surgical centres, because it is unlikely that such good results are achievable everywhere. Similar considerations may apply in future to studies which concern such techniques as balloon angioplasty and intracoronary streptokinase.

Another kind of problem relates to therapy which requires close supervision. Undoubtedly, the patients are more carefully controlled in trials than they are in ordinary life − more attention is paid to the toxic effects and, specifically in the case of anticoagulants, haemotological control is substantially better. This undoubtedly was an important factor which led many British and American physicians to abandon anticoagulants in spite of evidence in their favour. They felt that the marginal benefits demonstrated in the control studies probably would not be translated into clinical practice and that the risks of the treatment might then outweigh its benefits.

Another example of the quality of care being important relate to the success of resuscitation in trials comparing different forms of coronary care. Thus in the Nottingham studies on Home versus Hospital treatment (11), it was observed that there was no difference between the two, but it was also mentioned that no patient resuscitated in the coronary care unit survived. As the survival rate from cardiac resuscitation for ventricular fibrillation in most units is in excess of 50 per cent, this trial can be condemned on the basis of the poor quality of medical care alone quite apart from other considerations.

Another problem of concern is the care given to the placebo group in control trials. A specific example here is that of the placebo group in beta-blocking trials, strenuous efforts have been made not to give beta-blockade to patients who developed angina or hypertension and alternative therapies were given where possible. It is possible that such therapies (for example diuretic therapy) might indeed be harmful with regard to sudden death. Furthermore, it prevents the study being able to answer the question "should I be giving beta-blockers to all patients after infarction or only those who have angina and hypertension?", which is really what the clinician wants to know.

Who are the Ones that Benefit?

In almost all trials, and more particularly in those concerned with reducing mortality, the percentage of patients who benefit from the therapy is extremely small, seldom being greater than 10 per cent of the total treated. This certainly applies to the timolol trial (9), the European Coronary Artery Surgery Bypass trial (5) and the recent metoprolol trial (12), in which 3 per cent of patients benefitted. It is impossible to find out from these trials which particular patients have been helped, but it is unlikely to have been a random phenomenon. The clinician feels instinctively that there are certain patients who are more likely to benefit than others; this is an aspect of each of these trials which has not sufficiently been clarified. In the timolol trial (9) an effort was made to stratify by risk groups, but these probably failed to select those patients who were most likely to benefit from beta-blockade. Indeed, one can speculate that those who are most likely to benefit are those who develop angina easily or ST segments readily. If we accept the results of Theroux' study (13) in early post-infarction exercise testing, it is inconceivable that beta-blockade could have a significant benefit on those who failed to develop ST segment depression on minor exertion. In my view, therefore, it is not the correct deduction that one should give timolol or another beta-blocker to all patients after infarction but to select low-risk groups of patients for whom no therapy is called for.

How do you Equate Side Effects with Benefits?

This probably poses the biggest problem of all for clinicians, particularly in view of the previous point that the number of patients benefited by any therapy is usually quite small. All the antiarrhythmic drugs in current use have major side-effects, some of which are very obvious and others rather more subtle. Furthermore, the duration of trials is usually short but the recommended duration of therapy subsequently may be very long. Thus, while we can make remarks about the toxic effects of the drugs we use over a few months, whether there are adverse effects after several years is still not clear.

Conclusion

While the clinical trial is an essential research tool, extrapolation to the clinical situation has to be done with great care. The relevance of a trial depends on the careful choice of the hypothesis which is being tested and extent to which real-life circumstances are simulated.

References

1. Wilhelmsson C, Vedin JA, Wilhelmsen L, Tibblin G, Werko L. 1974. Reduction of sudden deaths after myocardial infarction by treatment with alprenolol. Lancet ii: 1157–1159.
2. Baber NS, Wainwright Evans D, Howitt G, Thomas M, Wilson C, Lewis JA, Dawes PM, Handler K, Tuson R. 1980. Multicentre post-infarction trial of propranolol in 49 hospitals

in the United Kingdom, Italy and Yugoslavia. British Heart Journal 44: 96–100.

3. Anturane Reinfarction Trial Research Group (ART). 1980. Sulfinpyrazone in the prevention of sudden death after myocardial infarction. New England Journal of Medicine 302: 250–256.

4. Multicentre International Study. 1977. Supplementary report – Reduction in mortality after myocardial infarction with long-term beta-adrenoceptor blockade. British Medical Journal 2: 419–421.

5. European Coronary Surgery Study Group. 1980. Prospective randomised study of coronary artery bypass surgery in stable angina pectoris. Lancet ii: 491–495.

6. Chamberlain DA, Jewitt DE, Julian DG, Campbell RWF, Boyle DMcC, Shanks RG et al. 1980. Oral mexiletine in high-risk patients after myocardial infarction. Lancet ii: 1324–1327.

7. Roden DM, Reele SB, Higgins SB, Mayol RF, Gammans RE, Oates JA, Woosley RL. 1980. Total suppression of ventricular arrhythmias by encainide. New England Journal of Medicine 302: 877–882.

8. Anderson, JL, Stewart JR, Perry BA, van Hamersveld DD, Johnson TA, Conard GJ, Chang SF, Kvam DC, Pitt B. 1981. Oral flecainide acetate for the treatment of ventricular arrhythmias. New England Journal of Medicine 305: 473–477.

9. Norwegian Multicenter Study Group. 1981. Timolol-induced reduction in mortality and reinfarction in patients surviving acute myocardial infarction. New England Journal of Medicine 304: 801–807.

10. Detre K, Peduzzi P, Murphy M, Hultgren H, Thomsen J, Oberman A, Takaro T. + Veterans Administration Co-operative Study Group for Surgery for Coronary Arterial Occlusive Disease. 1981. Effect of bypass surgery on survival in patients in low-risk and high-risk subgroups delineated by the use of simple clinical variables. Circulation 63: 1329–1338.

11. Hill JD, Hampton JR, Mitchell JRA. 1978. A randomised trial of home-versus-hospital management for patients with suspected myocardial infarction. Lancet i: 837–841.

12. Hjalmarson A, Elmfeldt D, Herlitz J, Holmberg S, Malek I, Nyberg G, Ryden L, Swedsberg K, Vedin A, Waagstein F, Waldenstrom A, Waldenstrom J, Wedel H, Wilhelmsen L, Wilhelmsson C. 1981. Effect on mortality of metropolol in acute myocardial infarction. A double blind randomised trial. Lancet ii: 823–827.

13. Theroux P, Waters DD, Halphin C, Debaisieux J-C, Mizgala HF. 1979. Prognostic value of exercise testing soon after myocardial infarction. New England Journal of Medicine 301: 301–345.

INDEX